Dental Ceramics

Ulrich Lohbauer · Renan Belli

Dental Ceramics

Fracture Mechanics and Engineering Design

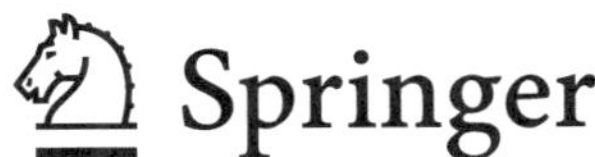

Springer

Ulrich Lohbauer
Dental Clinic 1 – Operative Dentistry
and Periodontology, Research
Laboratory for Dental Biomaterials
Friedrich-Alexander University of
Erlangen-Nuremberg
Erlangen, Germany

Renan Belli
Dental Clinic 1 – Operative Dentistry
and Periodontology, Research
Laboratory for Dental Biomaterials
Friedrich-Alexander University of
Erlangen-Nuremberg
Erlangen, Germany

ISBN 978-3-030-94689-0   ISBN 978-3-030-94687-6   (eBook)
https://doi.org/10.1007/978-3-030-94687-6

This Springer imprint is published by the registered company Springer Nature Switzerland AG
The registered company address is: Gewerbestrasse 11, 6330 Cham, Switzerland

Preface

Are there enough books about ceramics and glass-ceramics out there? Is there a sufficient number of books on the mechanics of fracture of brittle materials already available or do we need more? What about those subjects focused specifically on the discipline of prosthetic dentistry? Is the information collected in those books, updated? Is there room for new perspectives and new approaches to addressing the topic of the mechanics of fracture in dental ceramics, at all?

When we got confronted with the above questions, the decision to write this book fell heavily on the latter, despite the answers to most of them being dismissive of any need for yet another book on dental ceramics.

Our rationale here is to provide a dualistic perspective—yet not necessarily antithetical—on the fracture behavior of dental ceramics under several aspects: theory and practice, laboratorial and clinical, stability and failure. We go about it, for starters, offering some materials science background on the chemistry, synthesis, processing, and microstructure of dental ceramics and their relationships to the mechanical properties as assessed in a laboratorial setting, using the principles laid out by modern fracture mechanics. We confine the depth to modern, more clinically relevant materials, and forego on describing those that were once important, but that find increasingly fewer application in today's clinical practice.

Although undergraduate students of dental medicine and even dentists might find good use of much information contained herein, our main target audience was aimed to be the young researcher, that person who, as we once did, chose to take the path of academia, branching off from a typical career in the dental practice or in the industry, to pursue a profession oriented toward research and transfer of knowledge, both sedimented in a scientific concept. For that reason, we dedicate some space for digging into some of the fundamentals of mechanical testing and methodological approaches for determining material properties within a mechanistic framework.

In the last part of this book, we step out of the lab, yet not leaving the fundamentals of mechanics behind, to address the failure of dental ceramic constructs from the perspective of the forensic fractographer. By seizing on the richness of information that a clinically fractured prosthetic piece can offer on the fracture event, one can objectively address aspects of engineering design to reduce undesirable structural weaknesses and stress concentrations, thus guiding the way toward maximizing service lifetime. For that we employ the vast experience gathered in years of collaborative work in fractography courses and lessons learned from constant exchanges with renowned professionals and academics in the field of mechanical engineering.

We hope this book can generate some fresh perspectives on old problems and provide the reader with a basis for insights in materials development, a deeper understanding of mechanical concepts and incite the taste for accurate testing.

Erlangen, Germany   Ulrich Lohbauer
Renan Belli

Acknowledgements

Our scientific path up to the point of writing this book has been filled with extremely fruitful exchange of ideas with uncountable number of scientists in the field of dentistry and engineering, from whom we have learned a lot through informal talks and project collaborations. Our special appreciation for valuable insights and teamwork over the years must include the names of Susanne Scherrer, George Quinn, and Claus Mattheck. We also thank Achim Greß for his extensive help in producing much of the artwork in this book.

Contents

Introduction 1

Materials used in dentistry need to fulfill a certain performance in order to become indicated for an individual clinical case. This performance generally consists of demands toward biological and chemical stability as well as optical appearance and—most decisive—the mechanical resistance against intraoral loading. As materials for a restorative filling or prosthetic replacement are commonly in occlusal contact with the opposing dentition and need to function under load over time, the mechanical stability becomes the central property in dental decision-making.

This book aims to introduce the principles of fracture mechanics of brittle materials to the educated and interested readership with ambitious goals in dental materials science. The study of this book certainly requires background in mechanical basics and requires a sound analytical understanding of how to approach a scientific problem and how to simplify complex and multifactorial research questions. On the other hand, this book does not go that far to request a mathematical education or study of solid state physics. It is written for ambitious dental materials researchers from academia and industry starting their scientific path into deep and sound mechanical research on dental ceramics.

The structure of this book aims to introduce the mechanical principles of brittle materials and the underlying fracture mechanics concepts. The different practical techniques to approach the problem and the relations to material microstructure are of central focus, thereby supporting the fracture mechanics theory. Based on the description and characterization of the fracture process on the microscale, this book further aims to bridge and translate the knowledge to clinical reality. A complementary approach on defects and destruction and the implications for shape and construction design of dental restorations provides a holistic view on the clinical side and is follows a reverse engineering approach.

Bridging the gap between experimental observations, numerical simulations, and theoretical conclusions based on laboratory research with the in vivo clinical field application and related success rate is certainly the ultimate driving force of the book. Figure 1.1 shows the various levels of clinical evidence and the continuously simplified approach to restoration performance starting with wide scattered clinical assessments and ending with extremely standardized test procedures, such as measurement of fracture mechanics properties. However, based on those principal findings, the reverse engineering can start exactly here. The fractographic knowledge of the clinical fracture process together with the material response to external loading allows us to conclude on clinical indication, to experimentally and numerically predict clinical performance, and ultimately to recommend proper construction design and derive clinical preparation guidelines.

U. Lohbauer, R. Belli, *Dental Ceramics*, https://doi.org/10.1007/978-3-030-94687-6_1

Fig. 1.1 Reverse engineering approach from clinical application to material development

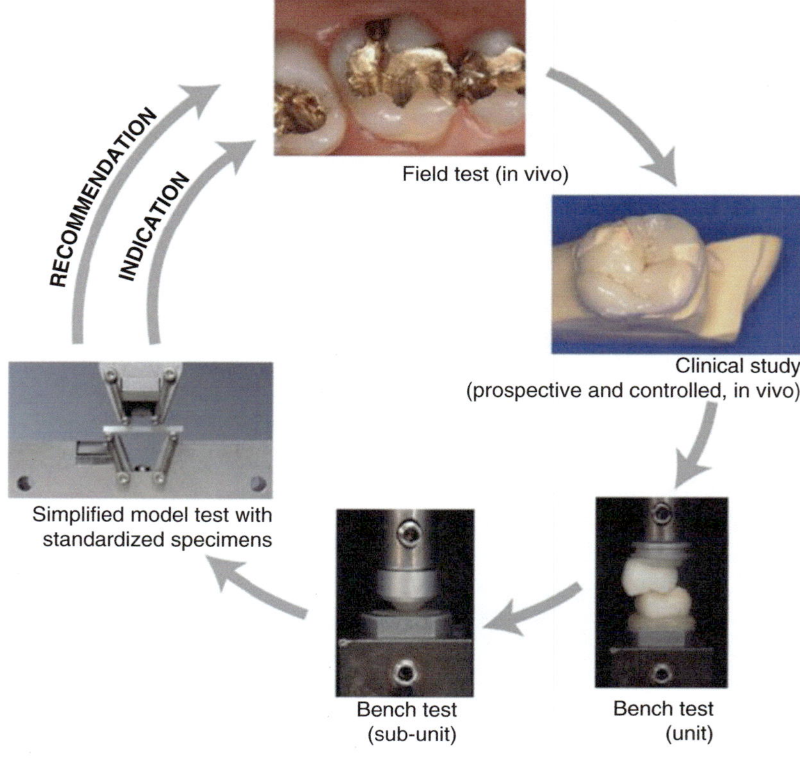

Chemistry and Microstructure 2

The effort to make sense of the broad assortment of ceramic-based materials available for dental applications can be frustrating, admittedly. This is more so for young professionals that have missed the train of development, which got momentum in 1980s with the translation of technical processing techniques to the dental field (e.g., hot pressing, CAD-CAM), which evolved rapidly by means of different material fabrication techniques, and is today at full speed, with new ceramics invading the market in an ever-increasing pace. In that sense, it is unhelpful for the clinician and laboratory technician to cling to product names instead of referring to materials by their chemical composition and/or microstructure. Not to lose sight of product brands is nonetheless advisable, once materials of the same type can slide widely across the spectrum of mechanical performance, depending on oxide chemistry and fabrication parameters employed by the manufacturer. Meaning that not every lithium disilicate product, for instance, is equivalent to some lithium disilicate that one might be expected to be referring to. Subtle changes in oxide ratios, particle size of the raw particulates, firing parameters, and so on, can lead to substantially different materials, including phase fractions, crystal type and shape, structural homogeneity, and internal stresses.

A simple way to classify dental ceramic-based materials is illustrated in Fig. 2.1, into three main categories: *hybrid ceramics*, *silicate ceramics*, and *oxide ceramics*. This terminology is not rig-orous, seen that *hybrid ceramics* here is naming scaffolds made out of glass or zirconia/alumina particles by partial sintering, which are later infiltrated by a low-viscosity polymer or a molten glass, respectively. The class of *silicate ceramics* is also hybrid in terms of microstructure, once they are composed by a SiO_2-rich glass fraction and one or more crystals types. Crystals can be crystallized from the glass following a nucleation and crystallization process (glass-ceramic process) or be added separately (particle reinforcement). Glass-free systems are contained in the class of *oxide ceramics* (though non-metallic glasses are also oxides)—which could well be termed "polycrystalline ceramics" or "non-silicate ceramics"—in dentistry represented by alumina (aluminum oxide, Al_2O_3), zirconia (zirconium dioxide, ZrO_2), and composites thereof. In Fig. 2.1, the subclasses are also distinguished whether by the specific fabrication technique (partial sintering, full sintering, or glass-ceramic process) or by the processing technique of the commercialized product (powder layering, CAD-CAM, or injection molding).

In this chapter, we will be waiving on historical fairness to attend mainly to the most relevant systems in modern prosthodontics, such as lithium (di)silicates and zirconias, with brief incursions in ceramic systems that find increasingly fewer applications, such as aluminosilicates (feldspar- and leucite-based) and hybrid materials (glass-infiltrated polycrystalline scaffolds and polymer-infiltrated glass scaffolds).

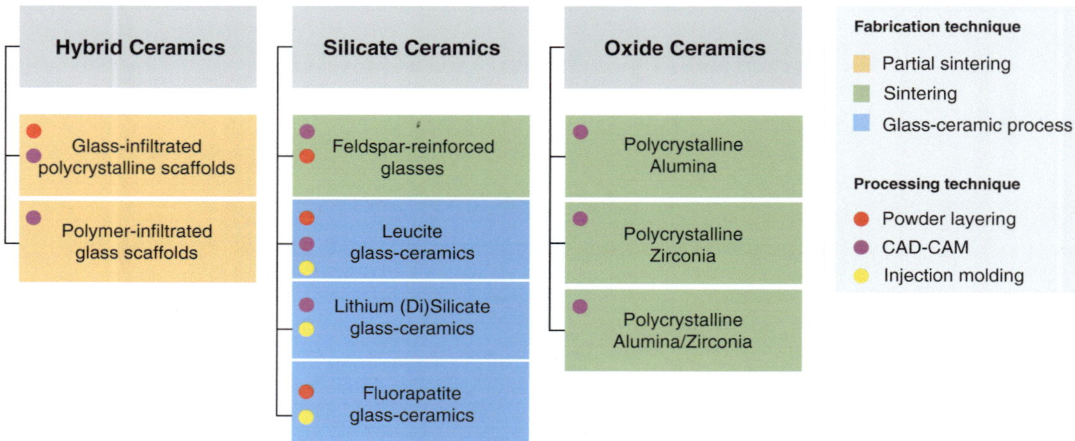

Fig. 2.1 A simplistic classification of dental ceramics based on chemistry and microstructure, fabrication, and processing techniques

2.1 Aluminosilicates

In dentistry, high-content Al^{3+} glasses are mainly of the tectosilicate family, having as alkali metal ions (M^+) sodium Na^+ or potassium K^+ in an Al/M ratio of 1, which compensate the deficit in electrical charge around the tetrahedral AlO_4 units, resulting in a highly polymerized glass network containing very few non-bridging oxygens [1]. They have been used for the production of dental powder veneering and machinable block "porcelains" via the synthetic route of glass-ceramic process or by milling natural feldspar rocks. The latter technique has been widely employed to produce the pioneering block ceramic materials for CAD-CAM processing, namely the Vitablocks® from Vita Zahnfabrik. The basic fabrication steps of this class are illustrated in Fig. 2.2, composed of the selection of high-purity feldspar natural rocks (usually albite $NaAlSi_3O_8$ and/or nepheline (Na, K)$AlSiO_4$), their milling into a fine powder, its melting and water quenching into a frit that is again milled for remelting and homogenization. To the powder resulting from the milling of the second frit, very fine milled particles of the original feldspar rock are added as reinforcing particles. Some products result from the mixture of two or more glass frits of different compositions and thermal properties. Those powders can be employed as a final prod-

uct for powder layering (veneering) or mixed to organic binders to be compacted, extruded to block shape, and sintered in the factory for use as CAD-CAM material. Feldspar reinforced blocks have a crystallinity of 20–40 vol.%, resulting in fracture toughness in the order of 1.2 MPa$\sqrt{m}$ [2, 3], with hints of a probable modest R-curve behavior [4].

In the glass-ceramic processing, potash aluminosilicate glasses crystallize leucite ($KAlSi_2O_6$), historically employed to adjust the coefficient of thermal expansion (CTE) of the veneering material to be compatible with metallic infrastructures [5], today also applicable as veneering onto polycrystalline ceramics. Bulk crystallization of leucite is induced by nucleation agents such as nano-sized leucite [6, 7] or Na-Ca titanate seeds [8], to form single or bundle of crystals, typically in crystal fractions between 10 and 30 vol.% in commercial products. The residual stresses and cracking around crystals that occur due to high CTE mismatches between crystal and residual glass, coupled with the cubic to tetragonal phase transformation of leucite taking place during cooling [9], seem to act as toughening mechanism in this system. However, although increasing leucite fraction leads to a linear increase in toughness up to about 1.3 MPa$\sqrt{m}$ [10], crystallinities over ~30 vol.% become deleterious to its mechanical performance [11, 12].

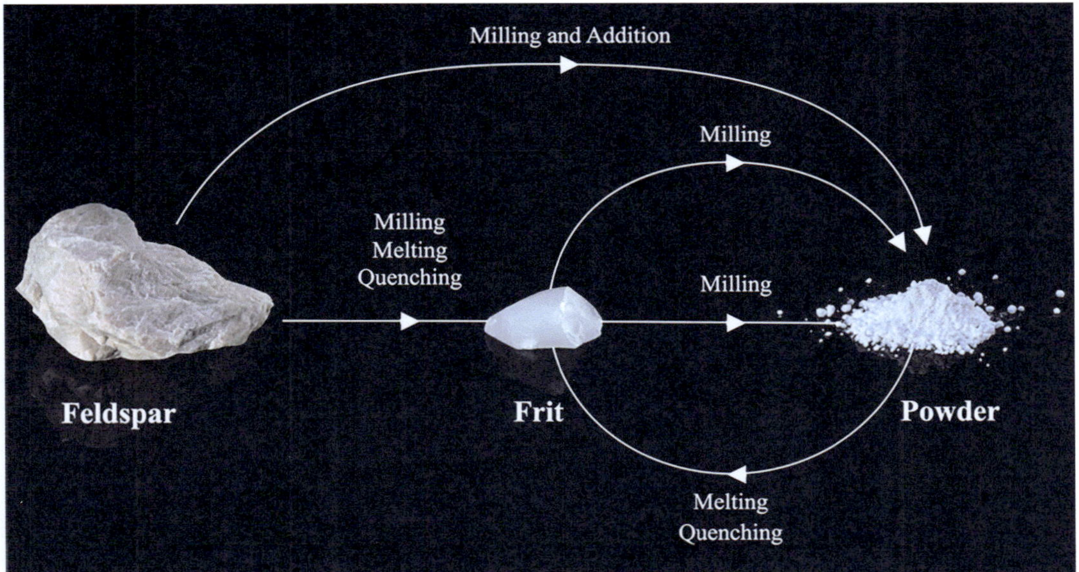

Fig. 2.2 Example of a fabrication route of feldspar-reinforced aluminosilicate glass

Although aluminosilicates based on feldspar and leucite have been important in the early development of all-ceramic systems, some factors have been responsible for the decline in their use in recent years, most importantly: (1) the increase in popularity of monolithic approaches that forgo the veneering step; (2) the advent of other highly esthetic veneering materials, such as fluorapatite-based; (3) the development of alternative techniques to veneering, such as the glass fusion or luting of ceramic overlays; (4) the consolidation of machinable lithium disilicate as competitor material having higher mechanical properties, among others. A testament to item (4) is illustrated in Fig. 2.3, where a higher fracture rate of leucite inlays and onlays has been reported, when compared to restorations made out of a lithium disilicate glass-ceramic [13].

2.2 Lithium-Based Glass-Ceramics

The importance that glass-ceramics based on the SiO_2–Li_2O system have on the landscape of current materials for prosthetic dentistry is difficult to exaggerate. Looking at the profusion of newly

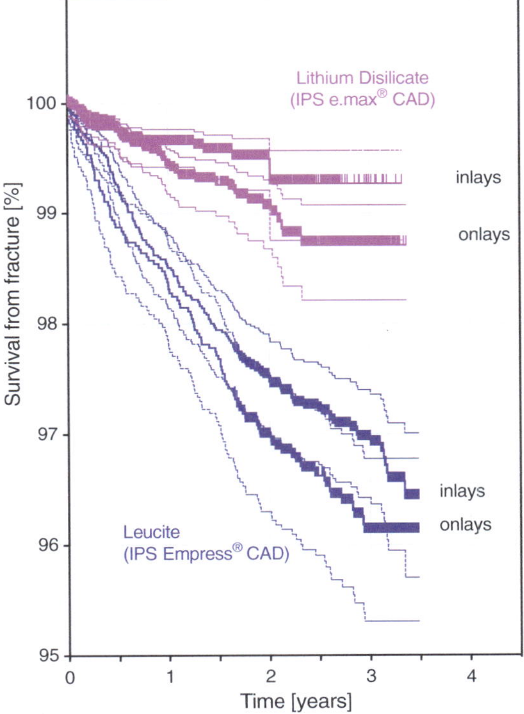

Fig. 2.3 Clinical fracture rates of inlay and onlay restorations produced by the same machining center, comparing the performance of leucite and lithium disilicate materials. From Ref. [13]

commercialized glass-ceramic products, with the vast majority falling under the enclave of *lithium (di)silicates*, one cannot escape to notice the silent operation of a *natural selection* type-of-process taking place in that domain over the last decades. This favors certain compositions to carry along their "traits" to next generations, while "unfit" materials are progressively dropped from the market. A similar phenomenon set the fate of the InCeram® product line, broadly used in the 1990s and early 2000s as all-ceramic framework materials, discontinued by the company Vita Zahnfabrik in 2015 after being over-performed by the newcomer class of dental zirconias.

Lithium disilicate, in particular, became a brand in itself, and its popularity is driving other glass-ceramic compositions to a rapid extinction. In today's dentistry, dominant traits are mainly mechanical and optical properties, with the fabrication route helping to tip the balance. For instance, the pioneering hot pressed injectable lithium disilicates (originally *IPS Empress® 2*, now *IPS e.max® Press*, both from Ivoclar-Vivadent AG), despite having superior mechanical performance and comparable esthetics [14], are losing territory to machinable analogs due to ease in processing, cost-effectiveness, and the *chairside* element. Also, psychological aspects imprinted in consumer behavior have their share in securing the survival or demise of entire product classes. For example, novel *lithium silicates* are surfing the same wave lithium disilicates gained by reputation, thereby conquering considerable market share by inertia, despite inferior mechanical properties. Conscious of that, companies have resorted to efficient strategies to push for lithium silicates, for instance by coupling specific products to their proprietary CAD/CAM systems, or shaping the branding to profit from the prestige of some of its composition (i.e., by using the slogan "zirconia-reinforced").

Unlike in biology, where natural selection assures biodiversity, the evolution of dental materials is sorted out by the invisible hand of the market, where economic factors set the pace. The consequence is being that the diversity within the class of ceramic materials available as dental restoratives is deemed to shrink. By the start of the 2020s, the assortment of products appears to consolidate lithium (di)silicates and dental zirconias as major players in the class of ceramics due to extended spectrum of use. Overlapping clinical indications, such as partial restorations (i.e., inlay and onlays), are up for grabs, with indirect composites competing for space. For short- to medium-range indications, such as crowns and 3-unit bridges anterior bridges, formerly confined to the purview of veneered infrastructures and lithium disilicates, are now claimed by monolithic translucent zirconias.

What is oblivious to the most ordinary practitioners is the fierce legal fight for a billions worth market that is in play, and lithium-based glass-ceramics take center stage. Companies not satisfied as bystanders of the commercial success of the lithium disilicate products from Ivoclar-Vivadent AG, and eager to cash in in the lithium hype, sought to launch products that could circumvent patent protected compositions and fabrication processes. That task becomes nearly impractical, considering the broad spectrum of oxide composition that falls under the umbrella of a single patent, and how compositions overlap among different patents. Readers are referred to a list of the most important patents involving dental lithium-based glass-ceramics, recently summarized by Huang et al. [15]. This has resulted in numerous patent infringement litigations, some of which have found resolution, with others extending over many years. While some companies choose the way of court battles, others yield to license agreements not to suffer from commercialization restrictions that come into effect during legal disputes.

2.2.1 Compositional Variations

Lithium-based glass-ceramics are not inventions of the dental industry. Early dental products appearing in the end 1990s stem from the tailoring of lithium disilicate compositions, such as the photoetchable lithium disilicate glass Fotoceram®, the first synthetic glass-ceramic material ever produced, discovered accidentally by Stanley

D. Stookey in 1953, when working at Corning Inc. A similar product fabricated by Schott AG is named Foturan®. A brief history of the early developments of glass-ceramic materials can be found in Refs. [16, 17].

At this point, some definitions and clarifications on terminology are necessary for subsequent comprehension. It is important to distinguish generalizations employing the term *lithium disilicate* from its accurate use referring to the stoichiometric parent glass composition, i.e., $2SiO_2 \cdot Li_2O$ in a 2:1 SiO_2/Li_2O ratio in mol% (nearly 4:1 ratio in wt.%), sometimes abbreviated as LS_2. Another common stoichiometry of lithium-based glasses occurs in the 1:1 mol% ratio of SiO_2 to Li_2O (approx. 2:1 in wt.%), or $SiO_2 \cdot Li_2O$, termed *lithium silicate* (LS). In glass science, stoichiometry refers to the glass and the crystal phases being isochemical, that is, having the same composition but differing in structural arrangement (crystal vs. glass). The crystallization of $2SiO_2 \cdot Li_2O$ gives rise to a glass-ceramic containing $Li_2Si_2O_5$ (lithium disilicate) crystals with a residual isochemical $2SiO_2 \cdot Li_2O$ glass, which can be crystallized to 100 vol.% crystal fraction, a slow process that can take many hours. Analogously, $SiO_2 \cdot Li_2O$ glass crystallizes Li_2SiO_3 (lithium metasilicate). It is therefore easy to conclude, that during crystallization the residual glasses in such compositions must maintain its stoichiometry.

Dental lithium-based glass-ceramics are not stoichiometric, but based on multicomponent glasses, where other oxides (mostly Al_2O_3, K_2O, CeO_2, and other trace oxides) apart from SiO_2 and Li_2O are added for purposes of decreasing melting temperature and viscosity, increasing the resistance to chemical solubility, but mainly to accelerate the crystallization kinetics by means of nucleation agents, such as phosphorus pentoxide (P_2O_5). Although there seems to be little convention for nomenclature on the basis of multicomponent compositions, *lithium disilicate* is employed informally for materials having predominantly the $Li_2Si_2O_5$ phase, with *lithium silicate* for those composed mainly of Li_2SiO_3 phase. For those materials composed of both Li_2SiO_3 and $Li_2Si_2O_5$, we have been using the term *lithium (di)silicate*, incognizant of more appropriate denominations. The vast majority of dental compositions also present some small (<10 vol.%) of lithium orthophosphate (Li_3PO_4). A list of main oxide composition and crystal phase fraction present in many current lithium-based glass-ceramics is given in Table 2.1, as determined by X-Ray Fluorescence (XRF) and Inductively Coupled Plasma-Optical Emission Spectroscopy (ICP-OES) [18].

The term multicomponent does not equate to being non-stoichiometric, which refers to deviations from the stoichiometric ratios of SiO_2 to Li_2O within the boundaries of this binary system. Multicomponent glasses can have stoichiometric SiO_2/Li_2O ratios, but that does not make them stoichiometric glasses. Early dental lithium-based glass-ceramics had SiO_2/Li_2O ratios larger than 2, while maintaining the SiO_2 mol% content around that found in the lithium disilicate stoichiometric composition (66.6 mol%). The addition of other supplemental oxides occurs therefore at the expense of Li_2O, invariably reducing the maximum achievable crystallinity, and resulting in a SiO_2-rich residual glass, which can favor the crystallization of cristobalite and quartz phases (both SiO_2) in some compositions. During nucleation and crystallization of multicomponent glasses, the residual glass is under a permanent change in chemistry and network structure (as opposed to stoichiometric glasses), making for very complex glasses that interact dynamically with the developing crystal phases regarding thermal behavior.

More recent lithium-based products show SiO_2/Li_2O ratios between below 2, or around 3. In the SiO_2–Li_2O binary system, the crystallized phases are tightly linked to the SiO_2/Li_2O ratio [19], as illustrated in the phase diagram in Fig. 2.4. The three colored areas highlight the compositions and temperatures in which Li_2SiO_3 and $Li_2Si_2O_5$ precipitate alone or combined. It is, in principle, inappropriate to project multicomponent compositions onto the binary phase diagram for purposes of estimating the solid solutions that may come to crystal-

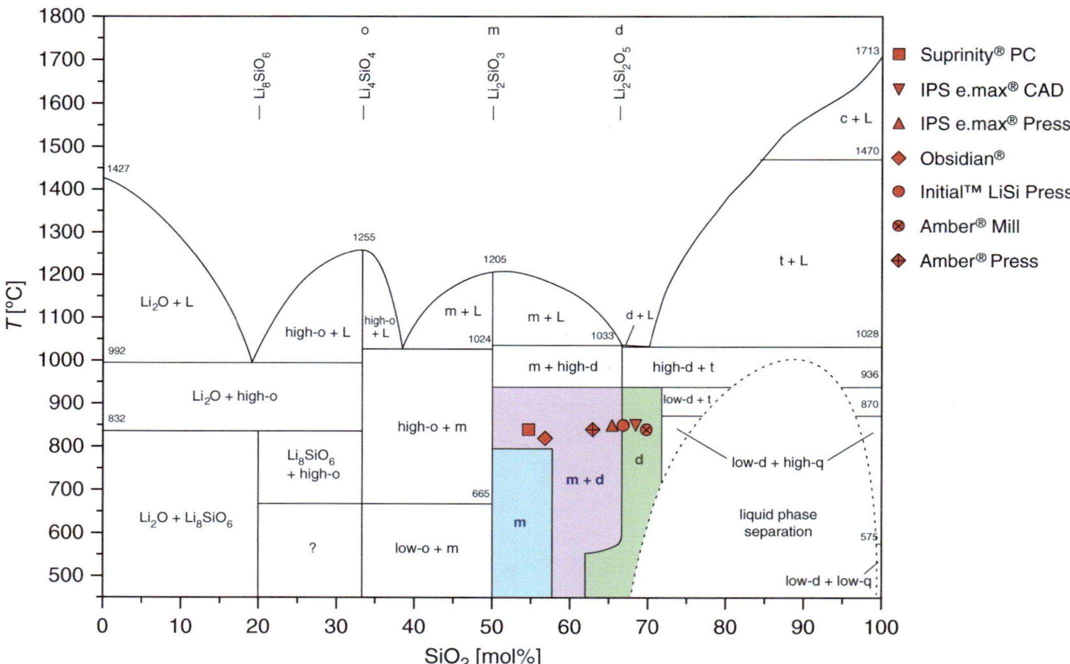

Fig. 2.4 SiO_2–Li_2O binary system, adapted from Ref. [19] with superposed dental multicomponent compositions

lize out of the parent glasses, whether using the nominal SiO_2 content or as a normalized SiO_2/Li_2O ratio. One sees that an attempt to map some dental compositions onto the phase diagram results in good matches concerning the crystal phases found after crystallization at the final temperature (compare to final phase fractions in Table 2.1). However, for some products it fails in assigning the final phases (such as for Obsidian®, which has no $Li_2Si_2O_5$ phase), as well as some phases in the pre-crystallized materials (such as for IPS e.max® CAD, in which $Li_2Si_2O_5$ transforms from a precursory Li_2SiO_3 phase). It is therefore evident the important role other oxides play in the crystallization of multicomponent SiO_2–Li_2O glasses, apart from the SiO_2/Li_2O ratio, particularly the nucleation agent P_2O_5. In such complex systems, the increase in Li_2O in relation to SiO_2 decreases the activation energy (lowers the peak crystallization temperature) for crystallization of Li_2SiO_3, increases its size, while shifting the transformation temperature to $Li_2Si_2O_5$

to higher temperatures [20]. Unfortunately, deeper investigations on the effect of SiO_2/Li_2O ratio in compositions similar to dental products with SiO_2/Li_2O < 2.5 are generally lacking. As a case in point, the material Suprinity® PC, which has a very low SiO_2/Li_2O of 1.57, shows only a partial transformation from Li_2SiO_3 to $Li_2Si_2O_5$, with submicrometric crystal sizes. The material Obsidian®, on the other hand, has a SiO_2/Li_2O of 1.88, but crystallizes entirely as Li_2SiO_3 up to 900 °C, with no signs of $Li_2Si_2O_5$ [21, 22].

Recently, zirconium dioxide (ZrO_2) has been incorporated in some dental glass-ceramic products in high amounts (up to 10 wt.% in the base glass—4.5 mol%) [23], and accounted for by some manufacturers to aid in strengthening the glass-ceramic. No crystalline ZrO_2 phase has been found in those compositions [24], with little evidence to conclude on any reinforcing mechanism. On the opposite, Zr^{4+} seems to enrich the residual glass phase as part of the glass network during crystallization. Actually, in $2SiO_2 \cdot Li_2O$

Table 2.1 Chemical composition (in mol%) and crystallinity of some dental lithium-based glass-ceramics

Material	Manufacturer	SiO_2	Li_2O	$SiO_2/$ Li_2O	P_2O_5	ZrO_2	Al_2O_3	K_2O	CeO_2	MgO	Crystal phases
IPS e..max® CAD	Ivoclar-Vivadent	68.3	24.3	**2.81**	1.33	0.37	1.97	2.42	0.83	0.24	60.3 vol.% $Li_2Si_2O_5$ 6.8 vol.% Li_3PO_4 1.0 vol.% Cristobalite
IPS e.max® Press		64.2	26.0	**2.46**	1.76	0.30	1.3	2.50	0.23	1.02	53 vol.% $Li_2Si_2O_5$ 1.2 vol.% Li_2SiO_3 7.3 vol.% Li_3PO_4
Suprinity® PC	Vita Zahnfabrik	54.7	34.9	**1.57**	2.31	4.52	1.13	1.14	0.65	0.21	27.1 vol.% Li_2SiO_3 14.4 vol.% $Li_2Si_2O_5$ 11.6 vol.% Li_3PO_4
Initial™ LiSi Press	GC	66.8	24.3	**2.74**	1.16	0.41	2.93	1.29	0.47	0.18	44.9 vol.% $Li_2Si_2O_5$ 4.9 vol.% Li_3PO_4
Amber® Mill	Hass	69.8	23.0	**3.03**	1.50	0.01	1.68	1.77	0.57	0.38	46.1 vol.% $Li_2Si_2O_5$ 6.2 vol.% Li_3PO_4 13.2 vol.% quartz 0.7 vol.% Cristobalite
Amber® Press		62.9	28.1	**2.23**	1.47	0.25	1.21	2.50	0.47	0.47	42.3 vol.% $Li_2Si_2O_5$ 7.7 vol.% Li_2SiO_3 7.9 vol.% Li_3PO_4
N!CE®	Straumann	63.2	22.8	**2.77**	2.42	0.25	6.22	0.30	0.33	0.25	28.5 vol.% $Li_2Si_2O_5$ 6.2 vol.% Li_3PO_4 41.7 vol.% $LiAlSi_2O_6$
Obsidian®	Glidewell labs.	56,6	30.0	**1.88**	1.12	2.53	1.62	2.66	0.37	0.33	36.9 vol.% Li_2SiO_3 6.3 vol.% Li_3PO_4
CEREC Tessera™	Dentsply-Sirona	59.6	28.7	**2.07**	2.28	4.75	1.56	0.80	0.66	0.74	37.7 vol.% $Li_2Si_2O_5$ 11.2 vol.% Li_3PO_4 3.7 vol.% quartz
Celtra® Duo		54.7	34.9	**1.57**	2.31	4.52	1.13	1.14	0.65	0.21	26.9 vol.% Li_2SiO_3 12.9 vol.% $Li_2Si_2O_5$ 11.2 vol.% Li_3PO_4

glasses doped with 10 wt.% ZrO_2, Zr^{4+} enters the glass not as glass modifier but as network former, thus polymerizing the network [25]. Zr was shown to increase the Raman frequencies related to the $Q^{(3)}$ and $Q^{(4)}$ species when entering the Si position, leading to a concomitant $Q^{(2)}$-Zr phase to separate, inducing the precipitation of Li_2SiO_3 as precursor of $Li_2Si_2O_5$ [25] (here, $Q^{(n)}$ denotes the tetrahedral units, specifically, Q refers to TO_4 tetrahedra being T = Si, Al with a connectivity of

$n = 1$–4). As a consequence of the bigger cation size of Zr^{4+}, ZrO_2 doping reduces the elastic constants of the glass due to longer Zr-O and Si-O bonds, despite the higher polymerized network. ZrO_2 added to lithium disilicate glasses also increases the viscosity of the melt [26–29] and shifts the glass transition temperature toward higher values [26, 27, 29, 30], as is expected from a highly connected glass network. Further effects of ZrO_2 are related to an increase in the nucleation rate of Li_2SiO_3 while hindering crystal growth, resulting in the spheroidization of $Li_2Si_2O_5$ crystals after transformation from Li_2SiO_3 [26, 27, 30, 31]. One must be aware that such effects cannot be disentangled from the initial glass composition, making for difficult generalizations.

2.2.2 Nucleation and Crystallization Kinetics

Stoichiometric compositions of the Li_2O–SiO_2 binary system (e.g., $xSiO_2 \cdot Li_2O$, with $x = 1$ or 2) are among the most exhaustively studied "model" glasses for purposes of understanding the fundamentals of nucleation and crystallization processes. In $2SiO_2 \cdot Li_2O$ and small deviations from stoichiometry thereof [32], the precipitation of the stable $Li_2Si_2O_5$ phase occurs following a homogeneous nucleation mechanism, despite the parallel appearance of a transient unknown metastable phase at the early stages of nucleation, depending on the heat treatment [33–35]. For such homogeneous nucleated glasses, the path for crystallization is taken to be:

$$Li_2O\,(glass) + 2SiO_2\,(glass) \rightarrow Li_2Si_2O_5\,(crystal). \tag{2.1}$$

To promote nucleation more rapidly, multicomponent compositions make use of what is called a nucleation agent, usually in the form of an oxide added to the base glass powder mixture. Common in glass systems are, for example, ZrO_2, Ti_2O, and P_2O_5, the latter being the most efficient one for inducing rapid nucleation in lithium-based silicate glasses. ZrO_2 does not seem to play the role of nucleation agent in these glasses, despite affecting how the crystallization progresses [30, 36]. In dental multicomponent compositions, P_2O_5 is also the main nucleation agent used, usually in a concentration from 2 to 6 wt.%. P_2O_5 is believed to induce an embryotic amorphous Li_3PO_4 structure that acts as epitaxial center for the so-called heterogeneous nucleation of Li_2SiO_3 [20, 37]. Increasing the amount of P_2O_5 has a decisive effect on the posterior crystallization kinetics, by decreasing the activation energy for crystallization of Li_2SiO_3, which occurs simply by:

$$Li_2O\,(glass) + SiO_2\,(glass) \rightarrow Li_2SiO_3\,(crystal). \tag{2.2}$$

This is a simplistic representation of the reaction. One must bear in mind that the unit cell of Li_2SiO_3 is composed of 8 Li^+ ions and 4 $[SiO_4]^{4-}$ tetrahedra, with two of their O^{2-} ions being shared with neighboring tetrahedra (i.e., $Z = 4$). With the two bridging oxygens, the Si-O group becomes $[SiO_3]^{2-}$ arranged in linear chains (inosilicate) along the (001) plane. Reaction (2.2) takes place usually between 640 °C and 700 °C in most dental compositions, which can be obtained from differential scanning calorimetry. With the increase in temperature, usually between 820 °C and 850 °C, Li_2SiO_3 transform in $Li_2Si_2O_5$ crystals by means of the diffusion of a SiO_2 "unit" at the interface, with equally $Z = 4$ for $Li_2Si_2O_5$, meaning that 4 SiO_2 units are incorporated per unit cell:

$$Li_2SiO_3\,(crystal) + SiO_2\,(glass) \rightarrow Li_2Si_2O_5\,(crystal). \tag{2.3}$$

The Si-O group is $[Si_2O_5]^{2-}$, arranged in two-dimensional sheets of hexagonal $[SiO_4]^{4-}$ tetrahedra (phyllosilicate) connected by three bridging oxygens, with the Li^+ ions connecting the sheets. The incorporation of 4 SiO_2 units results in a 41 vol.% increase in volume, with the unit cell of Li_2SiO_3 measuring 237 $Å^3$ and the unit cell volume of $Li_2Si_2O_5$ measuring 406 $Å^3$, a difference amounting to 71% of the volume of the Li_2SiO_3 unit cell. The structures of the unit cells of both crystals are illustrated in Fig. 2.5.

In the material IPS e.max® CAD, the difference in volume of the Li_2SiO_3 and $Li_2Si_2O_5$ unit cells were found comparable to the change in volume of the crystallized fraction after the second heat treatment [41], indicating thus that all formed $Li_2Si_2O_5$ stemmed solely from reaction (2.3), with no apparent contribution of reaction (2.1). This is mainly due to a more favorable condition in the form of preexisting precursor (Li_2SiO_3 crystals), lowering the thermodynamic barrier for nucleation (transformation). The second heat treatment of the pre-crystallized materials, sometimes referred to as "crystallization firing," unfolds differently depending on the base glass composition and the glass-ceramic resulting from the first nucleation and crystallization processed during fabrication. In Suprinity® PC, for example, the total fraction of Li_2SiO_3 crystals in the pre-crystallized block transforms only partially to $Li_2Si_2O_5$, reaching a plateau after 12 min at 840 °C. The Li_2SiO_3 phase in the pre-crystallized blocks of Obsidian®, on the other hand, undergoes no transformation to $Li_2Si_2O_5$, rather a skeletal dissolution around the boundaries of the coherent scattering domains, presumably triggered by the thermodynamically favorable condition of crystallization of Li_3PO_4 from P_2O_5 trapped within the large Li_2SiO_3 crystals. In the isothermal stage at 820 °C, the nano-sized single crystals grow by Ostwald ripening in submicrometric spheroidal polycrystals [21, 22]. The evolution in crystallinity during the second heat treatment for these three materials is illustrated in Fig. 2.6. The XRD patterns before and after crystallization firing are shown in Fig. 2.7. The change in morphology during the isothermal stage is shown in Figs. 2.8, 2.9, and 2.10.

Of importance during reaction (2.3) is the dynamic change in the residual glass composition and network structure. Bischoff et al. [37] have shown for a multicomponent composition with SiO_2/Li_2O molar ratio of 2.39, that the Li_2SiO_3 to $Li_2Si_2O_5$ transformation restores the $Q^{(4)}/Q^{(3)}$ ratio preexistent in the parent glass, resulting in a more homogeneous distribution of $Q^{(n)}$ and Li^+ species across the network structure.

From Figs. 2.6, 2.7, and 2.8, one notices that the crystallization of small amounts of Li_3PO_4 takes place parallel to the dissolution of Li_2SiO_3, suggesting that P_2O_5 might actually drain Li_2O from Li_2SiO_3. These reactions have been proposed for IPS e.max® CAD (Eq. 2.4), Suprinity® PC (Eq. 2.5), and Obsidian® (Eq. 2.6), respectively, as follows:

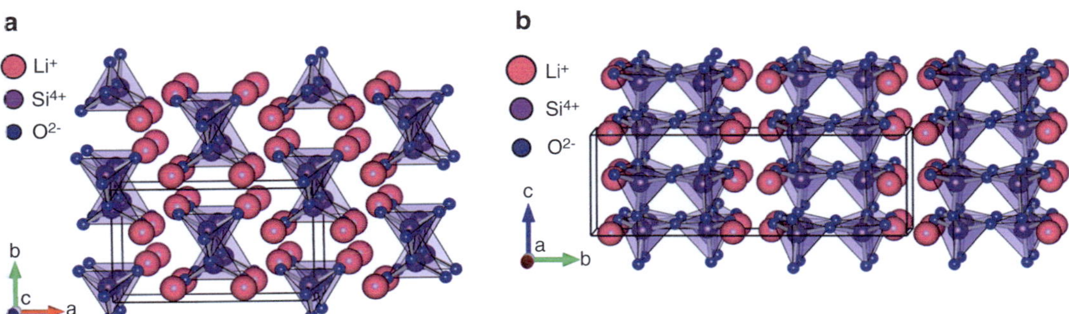

Fig. 2.5 Unit cell structure of (**a**) Li_2SiO_3 (ICSD #853, [38]) and (**b**) $Li_2Si_2O_5$ (ICSD #280481, [39]). Pink spheres are Li^+ ions, purple are Si^{4+} and blue are O^{2-}. Structure created with the Software VESTA [40] by K. Hurle

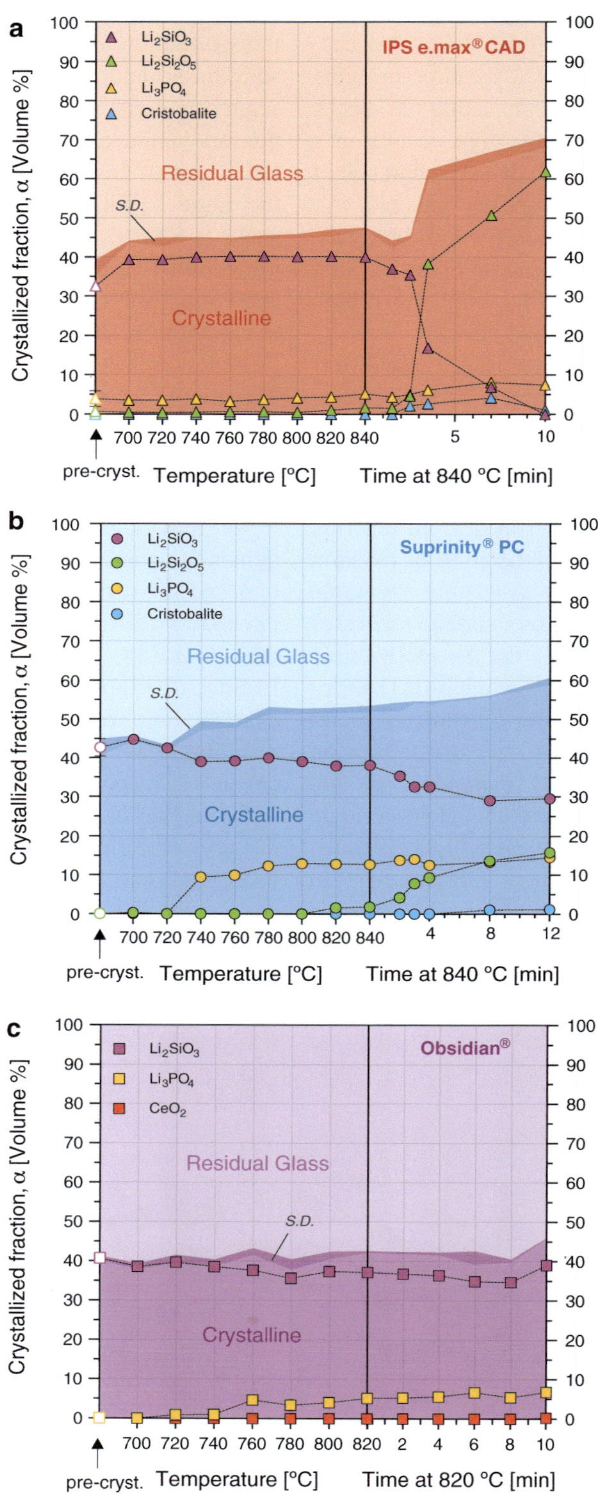

Fig. 2.6 Evolution of crystal and glass phase fractions during the "crystallization firing" of (**a**) IPS e.max® CAD, (**b**) Suprinity® PC, and (**c**) Obsidian®. Taken from Refs. [22, 41]. Reprinted with permission from Elsevier

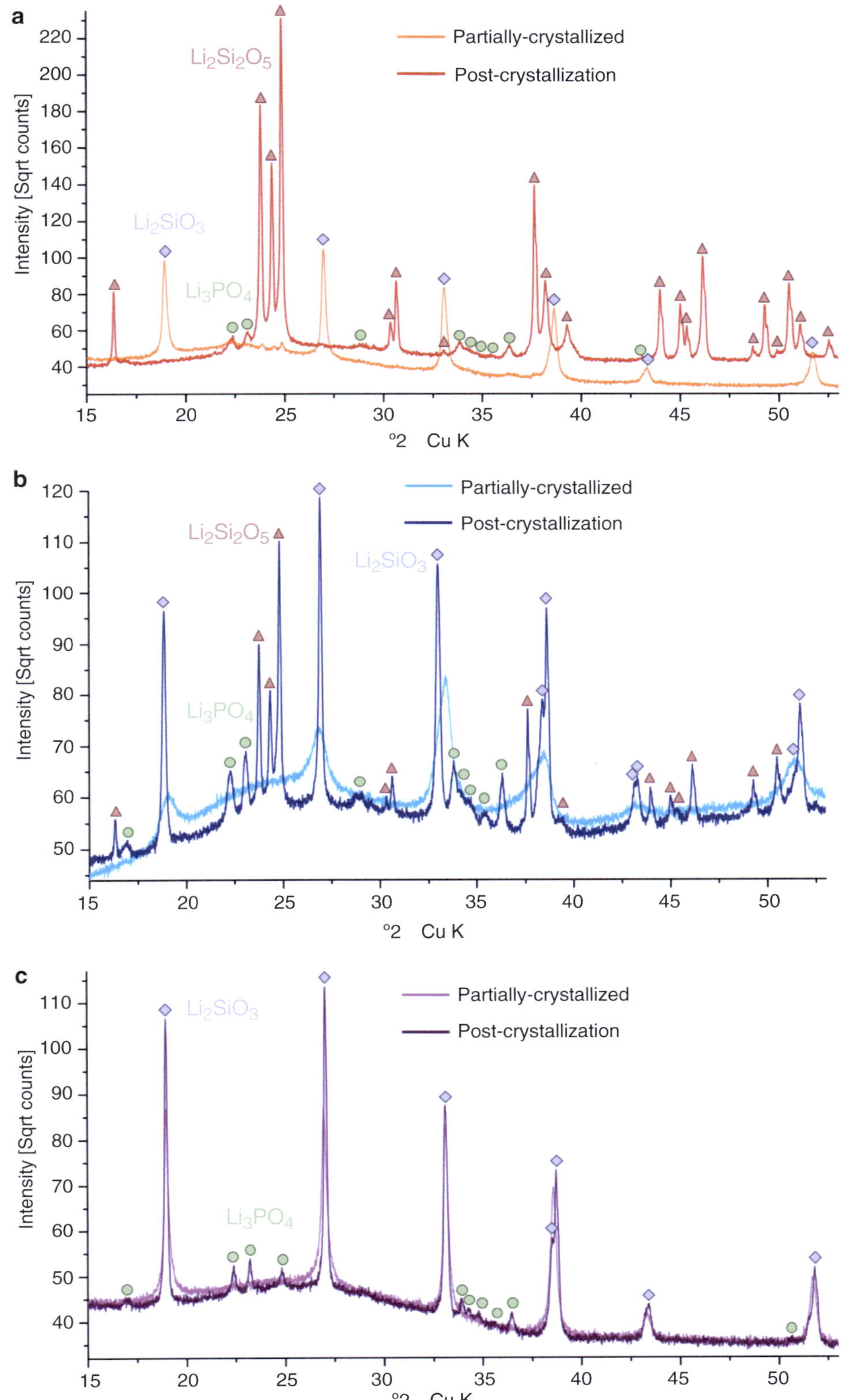

Fig. 2.7 X-Ray diffraction patterns of (**a**) Suprinity® PC, (**b**) IPS e.max® CAD, and (**c**) Obsidian® before and after the heat treatment "crystallization firing"

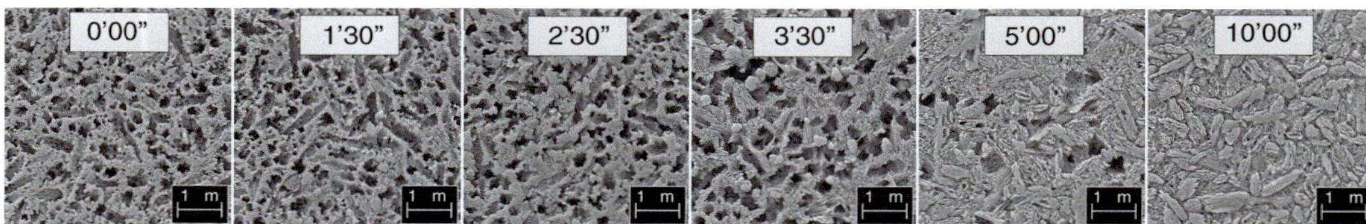

Fig. 2.8 Microstructural evolution of IPS e.max® CAD during the holding time at 840 °C, showing the transformation of each Li_2SiO_3 crystal (etched holes) in a $Li_2Si_2O_5$ crystal. Taken from Ref. [41]. Reprinted with permission from Elsevier

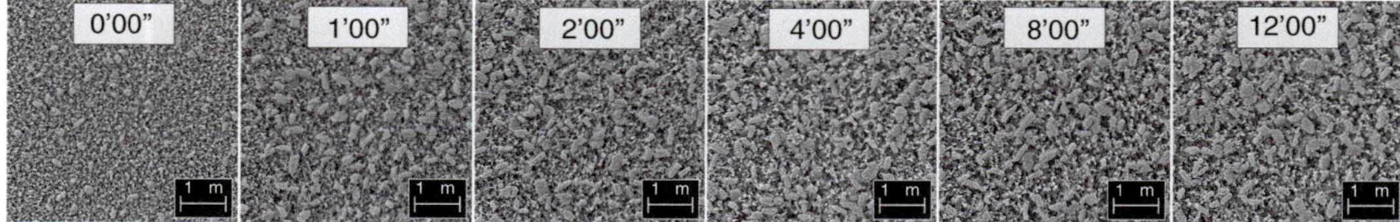

Fig. 2.9 Microstructural evolution of Suprinity® PC during the holding time at 840 °C, showing the impingement of newly transformed $Li_2Si_2O_5$ granules forming agglomerates. Taken from Ref. [41]. Reprinted with permission from Elsevier

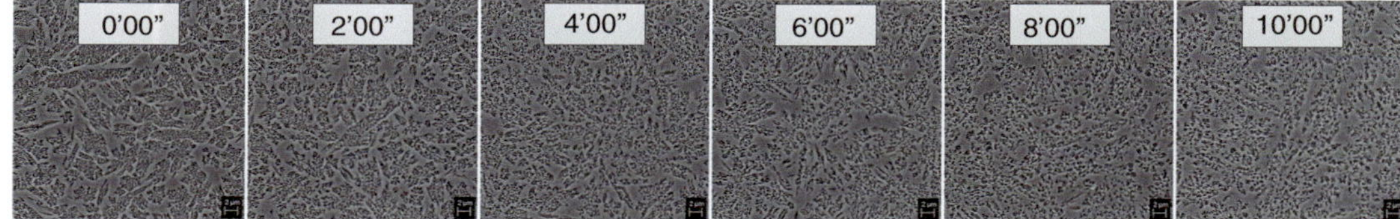

Fig. 2.10 Microstructural evolution of Obsidian® during the holding time at 820 °C, showing the progressive skeletal revitrification of the large pre-crystallized Li_2SiO_3 and subsequent coarsening. Taken from Ref. [22]. Reprinted with permission from Elsevier

$$3Li_2SiO_3\,(crystal) \xrightarrow{\text{dissolution}} 3SiO_2 + \left(3Li_2O\,\text{from crystal} + 1P_2O_5\,\text{from glass}\right) \quad (2.4)$$
$$\rightarrow 2Li_3PO_4\,(crystal) + 3SiO_2\,(crystal),$$

$$1Li_2SiO_3\,(crystal) \xrightarrow{\text{dissolution}} 1SiO_2 + \left(1Li_2O\,\text{from crystal} + 2Li_2O\,\text{from glass} + 1P_2O_5\,\text{from glass}\right)$$
$$\rightarrow 2Li_3PO_4\,(crystal) + 1SiO_2\,(glass), \quad (2.5)$$

$$3Li_2SiO_3\,(crystal) \xrightarrow{\text{dissolution}} 3SiO_2 + \left(3Li_2O\,\text{from crystal} + 1P_2O_5\,\text{from glass}\right)$$
$$\rightarrow 2Li_3PO_4\,(crystal) + 3SiO_2\,(glass). \quad (2.6)$$

Apparently, P_2O_5 can react with the by-product Li_2O from the Li_2SiO_3 dissolution, or with Li_2O if available from the glass. The higher temperature in which reaction (2.4) takes place for IPS e. max® CAD, favors the concomitant crystallization of cristobalite. In Obsidian®, the interstitial glass from the revitrification of the Li_2SiO_3 is enriched in SiO_2.

2.2.3 Mechanical Properties

In materials science, it has been sufficiently established that the mechanical properties cannot be disentangled from aspects related to the microstructure. In glass-ceramics though, the scope of microstructural effects exceeds the mandate of parameters usually responsible for making up for the mechanical behavior of polycrystalline ceramics, such as particulate properties (e.g., Young's modulus and fracture toughness), and geometrical attributes (e.g., particulate size and aspect ratio). The coexistence of two distinct phases (i.e., glass and crystal) gives rise to interactions that pertain to thermal compatibility, for instance. A higher linear thermal expansion coefficient (TEC) of the crystal will induce tensile stresses in the crystal and both compressive and tensile stresses in the glass phase, favoring a propagating crack to accelerate, or inducing microcracking already during cooling from the crystallization temperature. At low crystallized volume fractions, if cracking occurs, it is restricted to the region surrounding single crystals, while the overlapping of tensile zones in the glass may lead to microcracking distributed throughout the bulk material for moderate to high crystalline fraction materials. This has been observed, for example, for dental glass-ceramics containing high fractions of the Li_2SiO_3 phase, such as Suprinity® PC, Celtra® Duo, and Obsidian® [22, 42, 43], due to its high TEC of 15.4×10^{-6} K^{-1} [44] in comparison to the CTE of $Li_2Si_2O_5$ (10.1×10^{-6} K^{-1} [45]), in view of the TEC of the residual glasses in the order of $9\text{--}10 \times 10^{-6}$ K^{-1} [46]). For Suprinity® PC and Celtra® Duo, a high scatter in strength, in the form of low Weibull moduli, was attributed to bulk cracking stemming from such thermal incompatibility between phases [43]. Those cracks are present in the pre-crystallized material and persist passed crystallization firing due to the remaining high amount of Li_2SiO_3. The anisotropic nature of residual stresses that result from anisotropic TECs in highly elongated crystals has also been shown to impose significant loss in fracture resistance. A case in point is the observed toughening during crystallization firing of Obsidian®, which is believed to occur due to the spheroidization and isotropization of the Li_2SiO_3 phase [22]. In glass-ceramics composed predominantly by the $Li_2Si_2O_5$ phase, any thermal mismatch seems to be negligible enough for residual stresses in the crystal (compressive) and in the interstitial glass (tensile) to represent no harm to the structural integrity of the material, nor affect fracture toughness [46].

Particular to glass-ceramics, the degree of crystallization is the main factor affecting the final mechanical properties, especially fracture toughness, as shown for other systems [2, 10, 47, 48]. As a matter of fact, fracture toughness has been shown to develop linearly with the crystallized volume fraction, as shown for a stoichiometric $2SiO_2 \cdot Li_2O$ glass being crystallized from 0 to 100% with equiaxial $Li_2Si_2O_5$ crystals of 12 μm in size [49]. This relationship has been shown to be depictive of dental lithium (di)silicates during crystallization firing [41] as well. The toughening during crystallization firing is shown in Fig. 2.11a for three dental glass-ceramics, having mainly Li_2SiO_3 (Obsidian®), mixed Li_2SiO_3 + $Li_2Si_2O_5$ (Suprinity® PC) or mainly $Li_2Si_2O_5$ (IPS e.max® CAD) crystal phases (all having some low Li_3PO_4 content). In Fig. 2.11b, the relationship between fracture toughness and crystallinity seen in dental lithium (di)silicate materials is put in perspective to an upper bound set by large $Li_2Si_2O_5$ crystals in a residual $2SiO_2 \cdot Li_2O$ glass [49]. All dental products fall below this confine, for reasons related to other factors, such as crystal size and residual stresses. In Table 2.2, a summary of physical and mechanical properties, along with the average microstructural sizes, is listed for those products plotted in Fig. 2.11b [18]. The fracture toughness listed in that table was measured using a method based on a sharp surface crack in flexure, which circumvents the disadvantages of blunt notches, which tend to render overestimated K_{Ic}-values. Depending on the employed method, K_{Ic}-values can vary significantly, as exposed in a recent review [50]. It is therefore not uncommon to find in the literature higher values than those presented here; our values are in very close agreement with those from specialized technical laboratories and reputed authors [51].

One advantage of glass-ceramics having elongated crystalline phases randomly oriented, which can be achieved in both Li_2SiO_3 and $Li_2Si_2O_5$ crystals, in comparison to other axisymmetric crystals such as Leucite, is the ability to form an interlocking bulk microstructure that increases the spectrum of toughening mechanisms during crack growth. The fact that most dental lithium-

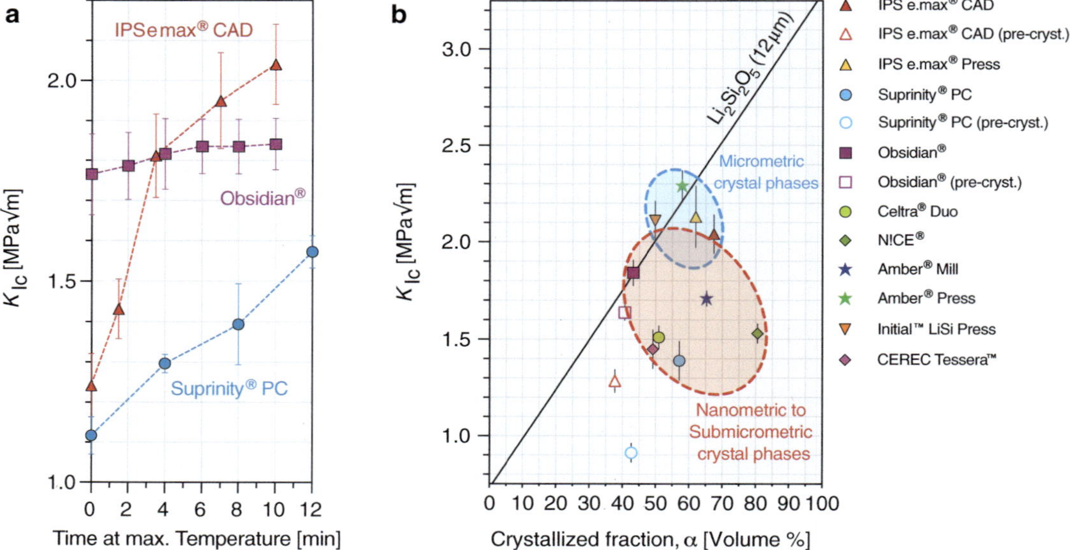

Fig. 2.11 Fracture toughness (K_{Ic}) of some dental lithium (di)silicate materials. In (**a**) the toughening is shown as a function of time at the maximum temperature during the crystallization firing. In (**b**) the fracture toughness of the pre-crystallized and crystalized materials is plotted versus the crystallinity in the context of an upper limit established by a stoichiometric $2SiO_2 \cdot Li_2O$ glass-ceramic with large equiaxial $Li_2Si_2O_5$ crystals. Image (**b**) taken from Ref. [18], reprinted with permission from Elsevier

based glass-ceramics rely on the $Li_2Si_2O_5$ crystal phase does not mean that it is a tougher crystal than Li_2SiO_3. In fact, a predominantly Li_2SiO_3 high aspect ratio plate-shaped microstructure has been shown to reach fracture toughness values up to 3.5 MPa$\sqrt{m}$ [52]. Such particulate shapes induce not only the typical mechanism in reinforced composites of crack deflection around particulates, but other highly energy-consuming cracks–crystal interactions such as crack branching and crack bridging. Resulting is the so-called R-curve behavior, common in materials having highly elongated crystals, which has been indirectly demonstrated for the material IPS e.max® Press, and to a lower degree for IPS e.max® CAD [14]. Especially in instances where a crack is allowed to grow for longer distances—in subcritical scenarios such as under fatigue cyclic loading—is where the R-curve contribution most counts. The extension of the lifetime of IPS e. max® Press by many orders of magnitude in comparison to IPS e.max® CAD, is a clear example of that, demonstrated in Ref. [53].

An advantage of pressable lithium disilicates is the ability to induce local crystal orientation leading to increases in fracture resistance [54, 55]. Crystal bundles oriented perpendicular to the growing crack plane have been shown to increase the fracture toughness by up to 25% [14], but also to force the crack into energetically unfavorable shear loading modes that increase the total (mode I + mode II) fracture toughness significantly [56]. Although this strategy is generally not practiced, the deliberate placement of the extrusion sprues in the wax-piece can significantly reinforce weak regions in dental constructs that result from anatomical design [57]. Pressable materials, unfortunately, suffer from substantial porosity, which tend to behave as critical defects and reduce their overall strength [14].

On the other hand, the practical disadvantage of machinable two-step materials (those which are machined and subsequently "crystallized"), namely, the need for special furnaces and the time-consuming heat treatment, is redeemed in terms of mechanical properties. The pre-

Table 2.2 Some physical and mechanical properties of some dental lithium-based glass-ceramics

Material	Young's Modulus [GPa]	Shear Modulus [GPa]	Density [g/cm^3]	Poisson's ratio	K_{Ic} [MPa$\sqrt{m}$]	Characteristic strength [MPa]/Weibull modulus	Microstructural size
IPS e.max® CAD (crystallized)	102.5	42.2	2.466	0.216	2.04	647.9/17.5	$Li_2Si_2O_5$ ~ 1 μm Li_3PO_4 < 50 nm Cristobalite ~ 0.1 μm
IPS e.max® CAD (pre-crystallized)	n.a.	n.a.	n.a.	n.a.	1.28	n.a.	Li_2SiO_3 ~ 0.7 μm Li_3PO_4 < 50 nm
IPS e.max® Press	100.8	41.9	n.a.	0.200	2.13 (random) 2.25 (oriented)	466.7/16.6	$Li_2Si_2O_5$ ~ 4 μm Li_3PO_4 < 200 nm
Suprinity® PC (crystallized)	102.9	43.0	2.604	0.208	1.39	611.2/5.3	Li_2SiO_3 < 50 nm $Li_2Si_2O_5$ ~ 0.4 μm Li_3PO_4 < 50 nm
Suprinity® PC (pre-crystallized)	n.a.	n.a.	n.a.	n.a.	0.91	n.a.	Li_2SiO_3 < 50 nm
Initial™ LiSi Press	102.9	42.4	2.435	0.213	2.11	n.a.	$Li_2Si_2O_5$ ~ 2 μm Li_3PO_4 < 200 nm
Amber® Mill	98.3	41.4	2.453	0.187	1.71	n.a.	$Li_2Si_2O_5$ ~ 0.5 μm Li_3PO_4 < 50 nm Quartz < 50 nm
Amber® Press	105.5	43.1	2.510	0.225	2.29	n.a.	Li_2SiO_3 ~ 3 μm $Li_2Si_2O_5$ ~ 5 μm Li_3PO_4 < 200 nm
N!CE®	91.7	38.9	2.629	0.180	1.53	n.a.	$Li_2Si_2O_5$ < 100 nm Li_3PO_4 < 100 nm $LiAlSi_2O_6$ < 100 nm
Obsidian® (crystallized)	100.0	40.9	2.622	0.220	1.84	n.a.	Li_2SiO_3 ~ 0.5 μm Li_3PO_4 < 100 nm
Obsidian® (pre-crystallized)	99.0	40.5	2.629	0.221	1.64	n.a.	Li_2SiO_3 ~ 5 μm Li_3PO_4 < 50 nm
CEREC Tessera™	103.1	41.9	2.622	0.229	1.45	n.a.	$Li_2Si_2O_5$ ~ 0.3 μm Li_3PO_4 < 50 nm
Celtra® Duo	107.6	44.1	2.623	0.220	1.52	626.8/5.2	Li_2SiO_3 < 50 nm $Li_2Si_2O_5$ ~ 0.8 μm Li_3PO_4 < 50 nm

crystallized state is usually less crystallized for the specific purpose to ease machinability and prolonging the lifetime of machining tools. But the lower degree of crystallization takes a toll in the fracture toughness, making them more susceptible to the surface and edge damage that must be sustained during machining. In feldspathic ceramics, for example, which have a fracture toughness of around 1.0 MPa$\sqrt{m}$, comparable to values shown for pre-crystallized lithium (di)silicates [42], machining damage has been shown to degrade the original strength by about half [58]. Polishing of machined surfaces can lead to some strength recovery [59], but it consists of a difficult procedure to perform appropriately and standardize in clinical practice. For two-step materials, the crystallization firing has been shown to heal cracks introduced by severe diamond grinding and sharp indentation pre-cracks [42], a process driven by viscous flow of the glass and capillarity forces. Polishing of the machined piece is nonetheless advisable, especially if conducted before the heat treatment. This is due to the smear layer of material debris covering the machined surface, which partly melts and forms a porous surface layer that act as fracture initiation sites [60]. The intaglio surface of constructs, rarely considered as deserving of polishing procedures, is especially at risk of such fracture modes.

2.3 Zirconium Dioxide

If one main accomplishment of the CAD-CAM revolution would have to be singled out, it could be argued without much need for persuasion, that the introduction of zirconia ceramics in dentistry was it. Up until then, infrastructure materials were fabricated whether by casting (metallic alloys), injection molding, or heat press/lost wax (IPS Empress® 2) or by slip-casting with subsequent glass infiltration (InCeram® Alumina/Zirconia/Spinell). The first two techniques require materials with relatively low melting points (for glasses a temperature between the glass transition temperature, T_g, and the liquidus temperature, T_L, high enough for the decrease in viscosity to enable extrusion). Since every prosthetic construct is unique in shape, a subtractive technique was therefore needed, which could, by design, machine pieces out of monolithic prefabricated blanks. CAD-CAM technology had the right credentials for such a task. Though the challenge to be overcome was the intrinsic disadvantages related to "hard machining" of fully sintered zirconia, such as long machining times and excessive tool wear. The solution came in the form of partially sintered materials with sufficient physical stability for thin pieces to be "soft-machined," nevertheless requiring a second sintering step to attain full density. Some hot-isostatic pressed (HIP) materials for hard machining have reached the market, but they represent a very small fraction of the form in which zirconia is utilized in dentistry; HIP processing is today mostly utilized for the manufacture of zirconia implants rather than prosthetic constructs by soft machining.

2.3.1 Zirconia Powders and Partial Sintering

Most of the zirconia powders utilized by dental companies for their zirconia products are preprocessed—supplied by few global chemical companies, such as Tosoh Corp.—and can be acquired in different compositions (i.e., Al_2O_3 and Y_2O_3 content). The raw material, in turn, used for the production of the primary zirconia particles in these powders, is zircon sand (zirconium silicate, $ZrSiO_4$) found in some costal sand deposits in varying concentrations. Among the many techniques available for synthesis of ZrO_2 nanopowders from the raw material, the most simple and cost-effective—and therefore widespread—is the coprecipitation route. The decomposition of $ZrSiO_4$ is achieved first by a fusion with alkali oxides, mainly sodium hydroxide NaOH (and eventually sodium carbonate Na_2CO_3), to form Na_2ZrO_3 and Na_2SiO_3. Hydrochloric acid is used in a second step for leaching silica and NaCl salt to obtain zirconium oxychloride $ZrOCl_2$, usually in the hydrated form of zirconyl chloride $ZrOCl_2 \cdot 8H2O$, to be mixed with a yttrium nitrate solution $Y(NO_3)_3$ at ratios depending on the desired amount of Yttria stabilization. Carboxylic acid solutions are used for the precipitation of zirconium carboxylates, for example, which render yttria-stabilized zirconia nanopowders after calcination.

The partially sintered blanks and blocks found for commercialization are usually produced by a double-stage pressing—usually by the primary manufacturer or outsourced to specialized companies—composed of a single- or double-action uniaxial pressing followed by isostatic pressing. The powder to be pressed is formed by the primary zirconia nanoparticles mixed with about 3 wt.% sintering additives (such as binders), resulting in spherical granules of primary particles having a certain size distribution. These powdered granulates are produced by spray drying, where the primary particles are mixed with solutions aimed to increase the pH (e.g., tetra-methyl ammonium hydroxide), additives (such as methanol solution of fluorochloromethane), dispersants (e.g., ammonium polymethacrylate salt), and water-soluble binders (such as polyvinyl alcohol, polyethylene glycol, and acrylic latex), to produce water-based slurries of well-dispersed particles having an adequate viscosity for spraying. At a specific flow rate, the slurry is sprayed into a hot air (~150 °C) stream chamber, where the moisture is evaporated from the droplets through the surface. Depending on molecule, the binder moves from the inner droplet and segregates on the sur-

face during drying [61–63], to form an outer shell that may affect the homogeneity of the green compact and favor sintering defects [61, 64]. It will be shown in Sect. 2.3.4 that the granule size distribution of the spray dried powders and the pressing steps have an enormous influence on the final mechanical properties of the fully sintered material, in special parameters related to the strength distribution.

The first partial sintering is a long-duration firing at lower temperatures (900–1000 °C), during which the additives are burned-out, and conceived to allow only sufficient mass transport between particles for neck formation. The resulting so-called "white-body" material reaches about half of the density and one-tenth of the Young's modulus of the fully sintered analog. In Fig. 2.12, different geometries of partially sintered zirconia blanks/blocks are shown, along with the typical appearance of their inner microstructure. Once these zirconia nanocrystals fuse (followed by grain growth), a linear shrinkage of 20–25 vol.% takes place, a dimensional change that is compensated by model over-scaling in the CAD software.

2.3.2   Phase Diagram and Crystal Polymorphs

If one tries to sinter pure zirconium dioxide, one will be successful in obtaining a dense monolithic integral material at very high temperatures, but be

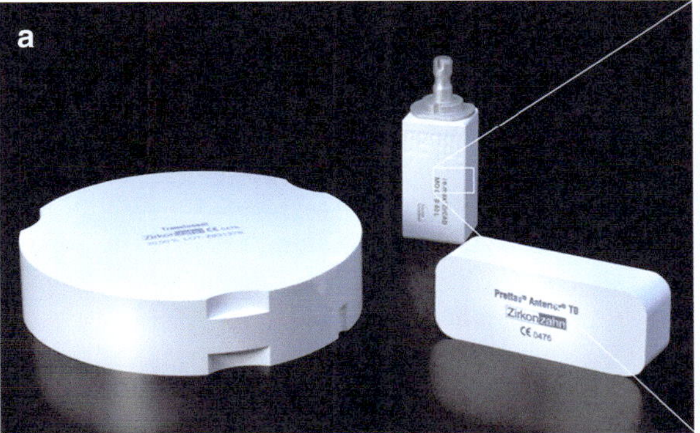
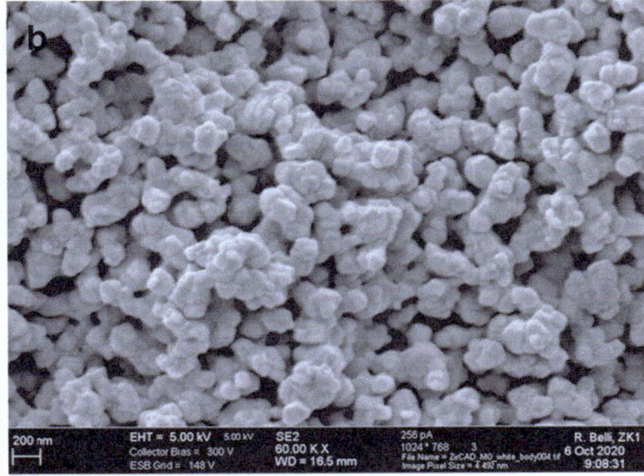

Fig. 2.12 (**a**) Blanks and blocks of partially sintered zirconia in different geometries for CAM processing; (**b**) scanning electron microscopy image of the microstructure of a white body showing the partially fused primary particles

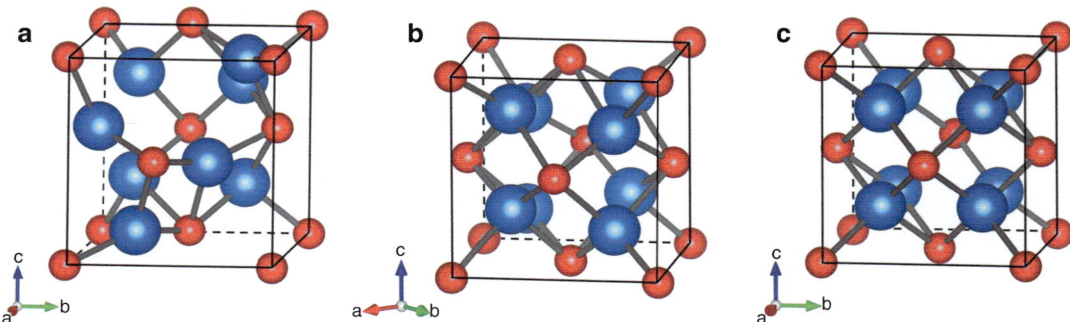

Fig. 2.13 The three allotropes of ZrO_2. (**a**) Monoclinic (ICSD #26488, Space group P2$_1$/c), (**b**) tetragonal (ISCD #90884, Space group P4$_2$/nmc), and (**c**) cubic (ICSD #89429, Space group Fm-3 m). Structures are created with the VESTA software [40] by K. Hurle

surprised to find fragmented pieces at the opening of the oven after cooling down to room temperature. This lies on the fact that the crystal structure of ZrO_2 undergoes changes in lattice shape along the temperature axis, assuming the allotropes monoclinic (*m*), tetragonal (*t*), or cubic (*c*), with accompanying changes in volume (see Fig. 2.13). The most significant change in volume occurs precisely when heating up or cooling down through 1170 °C, when the tetragonal structure transforms spontaneously to the *m*-phase (upon cooling), which is about 4.5% larger in volume than the *t*-phase. With this, high shear strains are generated inside the grains, leading to large stresses that culminate in cracking and loss of structural integrity. Because purely monoclinic zirconia has no impressive mechanical properties, coupled with interests in applications that demand exposure to very high temperatures—some even cyclic heating and cooling—where retaining the tetragonal or cubic phase would be required, extensive early studies on zirconia ceramic explored the potential of stabilizing both the *t*- and the *c*-phase upon cooling by alloying with other oxides, such as MgO (magnesia), CaO (calcia), CeO_2 (ceria), and Y_2O_3 (yttria). The most commercially relevant material for application in dentistry has been Yttria-stabilized zirconias (YSZ), originally in the 3 mol% fraction, which

stabilizes nearly the entire microstructure in the *t*-phase at room temperature, despite the theoretical stable phase being monoclinic; these materials have been termed yttria-stabilized tetragonal zirconia polycrystals (Y-TZP, with the mol% stabilization prefixing Y, e.g., 3Y-TZP). Relevant aspects related to dental zirconias have been recently reviewed in Refs. [65, 66].

The most accepted theory today concerning the fundamentals of an atomistic description of zirconia stabilization invokes concepts related to the local environment of the zirconium ions within the unit cell. It is believed that decreasing the "overcrowding" of oxygen anions around the smaller Zr^{4+} cations increases the stability of zirconia by the dilatation of the cation network [67–70]. This can be achieved by using "stabilizers" or "dopants" with a different oxidation state, such as the case of the oversized trivalent Y^{3+} ion, which induces an oxygen vacancy site within the lattice structure preferably located neighboring Zr^{4+} ions [71].

The crystallographic structures formed in YSZ materials are illustrated by the phase fields in the phase diagram in Fig. 2.14, as a function of temperature and Yttria fraction [72, 73]. The expression of Yttria content in the abscissa is commonly found as mol% $YO_{1.5}$, which can be converted in Y_2O_3 by:

$$Y_2O_3\left[\text{mol}\%\right] = \frac{YO_{1.5}\left[\text{mol}\%\right]/100}{2 - Y_{1.5}\left[\text{mol}\%\right]/100} \cdot 100, \tag{2.7}$$

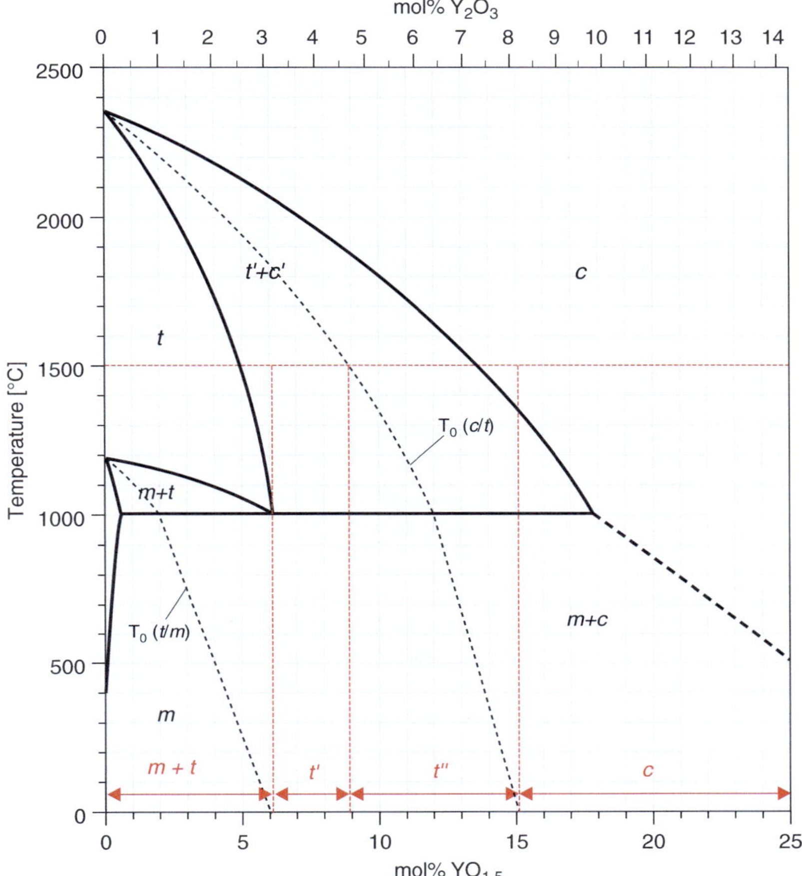

Fig. 2.14 Phase equilibrium diagram of the ZrO$_2$-Y$_2$O$_3$ system after Refs. [72, 73]. In red, the phases that are found after cooling from sintering temperature

projected on the upper x-axis in Fig. 2.14. Fully metastable tetragonal grains can be achieved by doping with as low as 1.5–3 mol% Y$_2$O$_3$ sintered inside the single-phase t-zone of the phase diagram. During cooling down through the T$_0$(t/m) line, the extremely low diffusion rate of Y^{3+} [74] hinders the partition into a Y-rich t-phase and a Y-depleted m-phase that would otherwise occur. Conversely, stabilization with >8 mol% Y$_2$O$_3$ results in a microstructure formed entirely of a stabilized c-phase, the so-called fully stabilized zirconias (FSZ). Stabilization of zirconias with Y$_2$O$_3$ contents between 3 and 8 mol% at the usual temperature of 1500 °C for dental zirconias, and the resulting phase composition at room temperature, are illustrated in red in Fig. 2.14. Bulk compositions between 3 and 4.6 mol% Y$_2$O$_3$ are located within the metastable supersaturated tetragonal field (t'), and stabiliza-

tions with 4.6–8.0 mol% in the supersaturated cubic field (c'). If these symmetries were to be kept upon cooling, the original t'-phase would persist at room temperature, while the high-temperature c'-phase would undergo a so-called *diffusionless non-suppressible* transformation to a tetragonal symmetry down through the T$_0$(c/t) line [75, 76]. If the available driving force for transformation is high enough, the high-temperature t'-phase undergoes a *displacive/shear* transformation mechanism in a twinned structure remaining t' at room temperature (the phase presenting ferroelastic domain switching [77]). The driving force being low, two tetragonal variants will coexist at room temperature, a t plus a t''-phase [78]. When transformed from a c'-phase upon cooling, an *ordering* of the anion sublattice occurs, resulting in a t''-phase that retains the stabilizer enrichment and a low tetragonality. The

t''-phase is non-transformable to the m allotrope, in contrast to the t-phase.

The Y^{3+} ion is known to show temperature-dependent segregation at high sintering temperatures, destabilizing the parent t' and c' in their metastable phase fields, into coherent Y-lean (Y_2O_3 depleted) and Y-rich (Y_2O_3 enriched) phases [79–81]. Meaning that the parent phase decomposes toward the equilibrium phases t and c, that is, a fraction of the grains moves left and the other fraction moves to the right along the x-axis of the phase diagram, landing somewhere in between depending on the time given. Recent studies on thermal barrier coatings having the same composition as dental zirconias have revealed that signals of a t' phase picked up by XRD consist of an artifact resulting from the interfacial coherency strains between the other two tetragonal phases, which gives rise to average lattice parameters [80, 82]. The coexistence of a residual parent t'-phase with other two tetragonal phases is, however, considered incompatible with the accepted theory of nucleation and growth, and thermodynamically inconsistent [81]. Phase fitting will profit from the inclusion of a t' phase on top of $t + t''$ patterns because t' reflections will remain resolvable in the XRD profile [82]. Similar artifacts tend to lead to assignments of a cubic phase in "translucent" dental zirconias doped with Y_2O_3 in concentrations 4–6 mol%, with c-phase fractions ranging from 20 wt.% up to 70 wt.% [83–86]. However, the presence of a cubic phase at room temperature for compositions <8 mol% Y_2O_3 is considered inconsistent with the thermodynamic understanding of phase transitions in the ZrO_2–Y_2O_3 system [72, 73]. X-Ray Diffraction is apparently less sensitive to perturbations on the anion sublattice (from where the tetragonality stems, see Fig. 2.13), exhibiting cubic-like peaks in <8 mol% Y_2O_3 compositions [79, 81, 82, 87]. When viewed under electron diffraction at TEM though, {112}-type reflections appear along the ⟨111⟩ zone axis, which are forbidden for the c-phase [79, 87].

Although these new evidences for 3–8 mol% YSZs regarding misinterpretations in phase assignments have been obtained for material fabricated by air plasma spray (APS) and electron-beam physical vapor deposition (EBPVD), they are supposed to be also valid for dental zirconias. In a TEM study of a dental 3Y-TZP, for example, selected area electron diffraction revealed only tetragonal peaks [89], even though XRD patterns in such compositions can be refined to include a c-phase [88]. Table 2.3 shows the stabilizer content (as well as Al_2O_3) of ten dental zirconias from five different manufacturers (including conventional and translucent compositions), together with a phase quantification considering the existence of two tetragonal phases and excluding the presence of a cubic phase. One notices that the increase in Y_2O_3 content in the bulk material leads to a decrease in t-phase with concomitant increase in t''-phase. The t-phase is more stable in Y-rich grains, with Y-lean grains being more readily transformable to the m-allotrope under mechanical stress.

2.3.3 Translucent Zirconias

Upon the realization that conventional 3Y-TZP suffered from considerable opacity, limiting its use in more esthetic areas other than as a thin infrastructure, great deals of effort have been diverted toward producing zirconias with higher light transmittance. The materials ensuing from those attempts are today assigned to different generations following an informal classification found popular in the dental literature, with 3Y-TZP containing about 0.25 wt.% Al_2O_3 belonging to the first generation. The initial strategy consisted of significantly reducing the content of the sintering aid Al_2O_3, which has a higher refractive index than zirconia, resulting in the second generation of 3Y-TZPs, though with negligible gains in translucency. The third generation has seen an increase in stabilization to 5 mol% Y_2O_3 under the rationale of increasing the content of an alleged cubic phase (a discussion on the unresolved issue regarding the assignment of phases in translucent zirconias is outlined in the previous section), which, due to its lattice symmetry, exhibits less light birefringence at the boundaries between the grains than that taking place between grains of the distorted structure of the t-phase. Additionally, this thought-to-be

Table 2.3 Chemical composition (Y_2O_3 and Al_2O_3 content measured by X-Ray Fluorescence) and phase characterization of conventional (3 mol% Y_2O_3) and translucent (4–5.5 mol% Y_2O_3) dental zirconias, considering only the presence of tetragonal phases

Material	Bulk mol% Y_2O_3/Al_2O_3	t (Y-lean) vol.%	mol% Y_2O_3	t'' (Y-rich) vol.%	mol% Y_2O_3
Prettau® (Zirkonzahn, Italy)	3.04/0.000	70.8 ± 0.1	2.47 ± 0.003	29.2 ± 0.1	6.12 ± 0.033
IPS e.max® ZirCAD MO (Ivoclar-Vivadent, Liechtenstein)	3.08/0.300	69.1 ± 0.8	2.38 ± 0.005	30.9 ± 0.8	6.46 ± 0.027
Cercon® ht (Dentsply-Sirona, USA)	3.12/0.049	69.0 ± 0.5	2.45 ± 0.005	31.0 ± 0.5	6.24 ± 0.012
Lava™ Plus (3 M Oral care, Germany)	3.15/0.111	67.7 ± 0.1	2.46 ± 0.005	32.4 ± 0.1	6.26 ± 0.031
Katana™ ML (Noritake, Japan)	4.07/0.112	59.3 ± 0.7	2.27 ± 0.021	40.7 ± 0.7	7.00 ± 0.025
IPS e.max® ZirCAD MT (Ivoclar-Vivadent, Liechtenstein)	4.28/0.050	53.5 ± 0.7	2.44 ± 0.015	46.6 ± 0.7	6.81 ± 0.007
Lava™ Esthetic (3 M Oral care, Germany)	4.84/0.113	41.2 ± 2.3	2.54 ± 0.020	58.8 ± 2.3	6.88 ± 0.011
Katana™ STML (Noritake, Japan)	5.36/0.000	36.4 ± 4.2	2.99 ± 0.145	63.7 ± 4.2	7.16 ± 0.033
Cercon® xt (Dentsply-Sirona, USA)	5.38/0.063	33.1 ± 0.3	2.95 ± 0.035	66.9 ± 0.3	7.08 ± 0.001
Prettau® Anterior (Zirkonzahn, Italy)	5.40/0.063	37.1 ± 4.8	3.10 ± 0.209	62.9 ± 4.8	7.01 ± 0.048

The amount of Y_2O_3 in each tetragonal phase is calculated based on the lattice parameters. Results from [88]

cubic phase grows into larger grains, which reduces the relative surface of grain boundaries where light scattering takes place. That third generation has seen a severe drop in mechanical performance [84, 86], as expected from the reduction on vol% fraction of the transformable t-phase. A backpedal was underway for the fourth generation in the form of a slight reduction in the Y_2O_3 content to 4 mol%, aimed at recovering some of the lost strength and toughness, thereby sacrificing translucency as well. It is spoken of a "trade-off" [90] between mechanical and optical properties, once aspects favoring one are poised to affect the other negatively. Increasing the amount of a less anisotropic phase (be that a cubic or a low-tetragonality t''-phase) takes a toll on the fracture toughness since less transformable volume is available to toughen the crack path. Increasing the grain size of t-phase can only be pursued up to a threshold grain size of about 1–2 μm [91] before spontaneous transformation to the m-phase gets in the way. Figure 2.15 shows the relationship between fracture toughness and stabilizer content in currently commercialized dental 3 mol%-, 4 mol%-, and 5 mol%-Y_2O_3-stabilized zirconias.

The most promising strategy to increase the translucency of predominantly tetragonal zirconias consists of exploiting the microstructural interactions with light by means of significantly reducing light scattering, namely by decreasing the grain size to the nanometric range ($\leq$100 nm) [92]. To achieve such a microstructure means solving several practical challenges that span from powder processing techniques up to sintering concepts, which seem to keep researchers and manufacturers currently occupied. Meanwhile, innovations in commercial products revolve around producing graded zirconias, whether by changing the pigmentation along the thickness of the machinable blank/block, or by structuring these blank/blocks with different layers of powders with varying concentrations of Y_2O_3, with a thickness gradient from 5 mol% to 3 mol% aiming to provide an enamel-to-dentin-like transition of color and translucency.

Fig. 2.15 Power–law relationship between K_{Ic} and Y_2O_3 content using a poll of literature data using sharp cracks (colored symbols, red regression) and using the CNB method (black circles, black regression). Data from Ref. [88]. Reprinted with permission from Elsevier

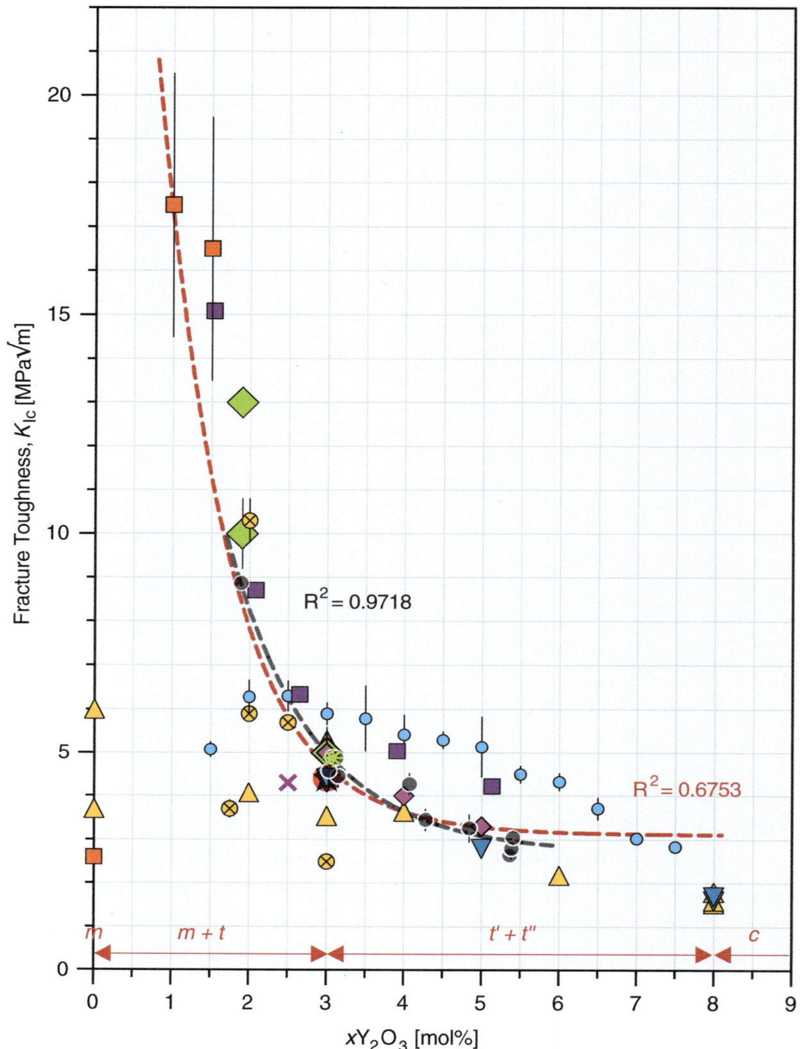

2.3.4 Mechanical Properties

The application of zirconia materials for use as a structural component, such as for orthopedic implants and dental prosthetics, could only have been so widespread today thank its excellent mechanical performance. Ferroelastic domain switching, the temperature-insensitive toughening mechanism in thermal barrier zirconia coatings containing the t'-phase [77], has no relevance for dental zirconias. Toughening of dental zirconias is mostly due to the metastability of the t-phase, which makes tetragonal grains suscepti-

ble to transformation to the stable m-phase upon localized stress concentration at the front of critical defects or cracks. The volume increase in the newly m-transformed grains induces high compressive stresses within a process zone ahead of the crack tip, which has to be overcome for the crack to grow. In terms of stress intensity factor, the now critical K_{appl}-value, K_{Ic}, is composed of the intrinsic K-value of the matrix (untransformable tetragonal phase), $K_{I,matrix}$, and the (negative) shielding K due to transformation, $K_{I,sh}$:

$$K_{Ic} = K_{I,matrix} - K_{I,sh}, \tag{2.8}$$

the last term being the so-called *transformation toughening* mechanism, which is alleged to be composed of a dilatational and a deviatoric component of strain [93]. Because dental zirconias exhibit a submicrometric grain-sized microstructure, specimen preparation for fracture toughness testing using sawed notches tend to produce excessively wide notch-root radii, which induce the overestimation of the true K_{Ic}. To circumvent the difficulty in producing atomically sharp cracks in zirconias, Chevron-notched beams (CNB) have been advised as an appropriate method due to the pop-in crack inherent of the specimen and loading geometry [50, 94]. In Fig. 2.15 the black circles represent values of K_{Ic} measured using the CNB method for a variety of conventional and translucent zirconias, including a technical 2Y-TZP for comparison. Single values for dental commercial products are listed in the last column of Table 2.4.

Traditionally, the relationship between K_{Ic} and Y_2O_3 fraction in YSZs has been based on the work of Lange [91] (see blue circles in Fig. 2.15), with new attempts showing a power–law relationship with high increments taking place at low stabilizations, between 1 and 3 MPa$\sqrt{m}$, following rather the tendency measured by Miyazaki [95] (purple squares in Fig. 2.15). If extrapolated toward high Y_2O_3 fractions containing low amounts of the transformable t-phase, the $K_{I,matrix}$ is expected to amount to 2–2.5 MPa$\sqrt{m}$, meaning that $K_{I,sh}$ would reach up to 2.5–3 MPa$\sqrt{m}$ for conventional dental 3Y-TZPs, and only 0.5–1 MPa$\sqrt{m}$ for translucent dental 5Y-TZPs. In that range of 3–5 mol% Y_2O_3 stabilization, K_{Ic} has a practically linear dependency on the t'-phase content [88]. For comparison, 4Y-TZPs for thermal barrier coating produced by EBPVD having t'-phase with predominantly ferroelastic domain switching exhibit a K_{Ic} of ~3 MPa$\sqrt{m}$ [96]. Interestingly, it has been found that not all the transformable t-grains at the crack path will transform, but a fraction thereof; the t-phase transformability gets diminished as the Y_2O_3 content increases [97, 98]. The transformation toughening is responsible for increasing the crack tip stress intensity factor as per Eq. (2.8), but conversely to zirconias stabilized with MgO, for example, the dependency on crack extension is

Table 2.4 Weibull characteristic strength σ_0 and modulus m [90% Confidence Interval] for two specimen sizes of conventional and translucent dental zirconias, with corresponding fracture toughness K_{Ic} ± Standard Deviation

Material	4 PB 4 × 3 mm²		B3B t = 1.2 mm		K_{Ic}
	σ_0 (MPa)	m	σ_0 (MPa)	m	(MPa$\sqrt{m}$)
Prettau®	1030.7 [1003–1059]	11.1 [8.9–14.0]	1273.2 [1249–1297]	17.0 [13.4–21.5]	4.57 ± 0.39
IPS e.max® ZirCAD MO	1071.5 [1054–1089]	18.2 [14.5–22.9]	1253.9 [1209–1300]	9.0 [7.1–11.4]	4.90 ± 0.19
Cercon® ht	1137.1 [1112–1169]	13.6 [10.8–17.1]	1246.2 [1224–1268]	18.6 [14.7–23.5]	4.87 ± 0.16
Lava™ Plus	1121.7 [1070–1176]	6.3 [5.1–8.0]	1336.7 [1272–1404]	6.6 [5.2–8.4]	4.45 ± 0.26
Katana™ ML	965.6 [934–998]	9.1 [7.3–11.5]	1248.9 [1216–1283]	12.1 [9.6–15.4]	4.27 ± 0.25
IPS e.max® ZirCAD MT	801.5 [780–823]	11.3 [9.0–14.2]	754.2 [714–797]	5.9 [4.6–7.4]	3.45 ± 0.24
Lava™ Esthetic	640.9 [615–667]	7.5 [6.0–9.4]	829.9 [779–883]	5.2 [4.1–6.6]	3.26 ± 0.31
Katana™ STML	622.6 [600–646]	8.1 [6.5–10.2]	744.1 [727–761]	13.9 [11.0–17.5]	2.64 ± 0.14
Cercon® xt	629.1 [613–645]	12.0 [9.5–15.1]	832.6 [800–866]	8.2 [6.5–10.3]	2.80 ± 0.23
Prettau® Anterior	625.6 [609–642]	11.3 [9.0–14.1]	761.5 [724–800]	6.5 [5.1–8.2]	3.05 ± 0.13

4 PB 4 × 3 mm² = Four-point bending with specimens having *width* × *height* of 4 × 3 mm² cross-section and 10/20 mm span lengths
B3B t = 1.2 mm = Ball-on-three-balls biaxial flexural strength with rectangular specimens having 1.2 mm in thickness
From Ref. [100]

apparently small in 3Y-TZPs, inducing very shallow R-curves [93, 99].

The relationship between fracture toughness and applied stress, as will be later established in Eq. (3.6) in Sect. 3.2.1, indicates that the fracture strength is inversely proportional to square root of the critical defect in the specimen, with a set of specimens showing a certain scatter depending on the defect size distribution in the material, as discussed in Sect. 3.1. As in any monolithic ceramic material, the high strength achieved in zirconia components—a material property which is much easier to be digested in terms of service load—cannot, therefore, be single-handedly due to its high fracture toughness, but by decreasing the size of defects in the sintered material. It becomes therefore of fundamental importance to identify the type and source of defects that are typical for a specific material, a task that usually leads one back to evaluate all the processing steps during production so to act on eliminating or reducing the size of defects that become critical at different relevant volumes in service. In machinable dental zirconias, it has been repeatedly demonstrated that the nature of critical defects can be traced back to the compaction of the powder [101, 102], resulting in fine elongated voids after sintering. Figure 2.16 shows one such defect in the partially sintered white body and it surviving the final sintering. Their presence in the white body indicates that they must have been present in the green body after cold-isostatic pressing too. They are formed mostly at the junction of several granules due to the inability of the primary particles therein to flow and fill all that space [103], probably due to the stiff segregated binder shell that is typical of spray-dried zirconia powders [61–63].

Conventional 3Y-TZPs are known to achieve flexural strength values >1000 MPa—a value that is of course dependent on the size of the tested specimen (See Sect. 3.1). In Table 2.4, the strength of dental zirconias stabilized with 3–5.4 mol% Y_2O_3, the same commercial products as in Table 2.3, is given for two specimen sizes having effective surfaces and volumes analogous to a small restoration (single crown) and a larger construct such as a 4-unit posterior bridge. As expected, the larger the size, the lower the strength. The reliability represented by the Weibull modulus m varies in a wide range from 5 up to 18, even within the same manufacturer. The increase in Y_2O_3 content can be seen to reduce the strength substantially, thus narrowing clinical applicability for translucent zirconias. In that respect, the decrease in strength is solely due to the lower K_{Ic} of the more stabilized YSZs, due to the fact that an equivalent defect size distribution seems to be present in most materials [100]. That indicates that most manufacturers are using feedstocks that stem from a small number of powder providers, or that granulate size distributions are

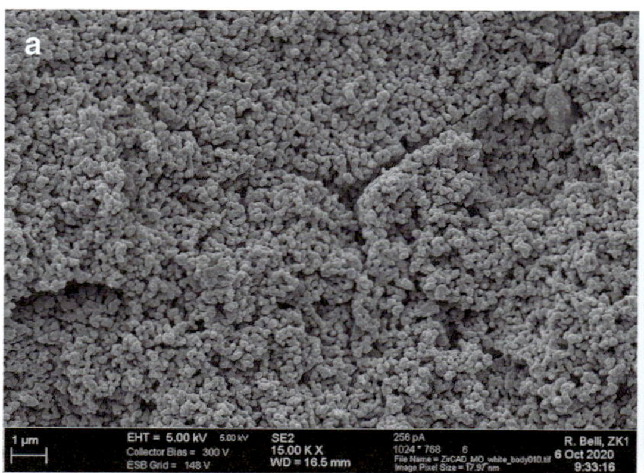
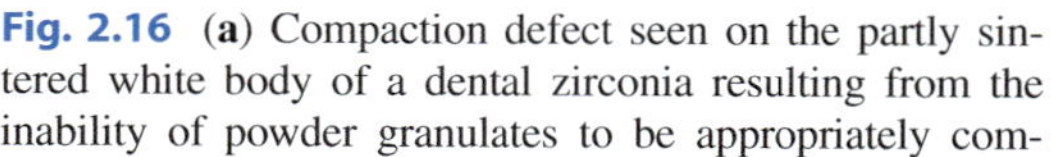
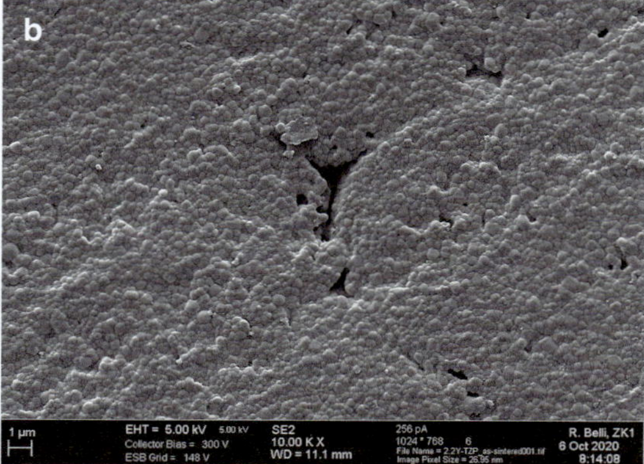

Fig. 2.16 (**a**) Compaction defect seen on the partly sintered white body of a dental zirconia resulting from the inability of powder granulates to be appropriately compacted at their junctions (from Ref. [100]). Reprinted with permission from Elsevier. These defects are not healed during sintering, resulting in voids as the one observed in (**b**)

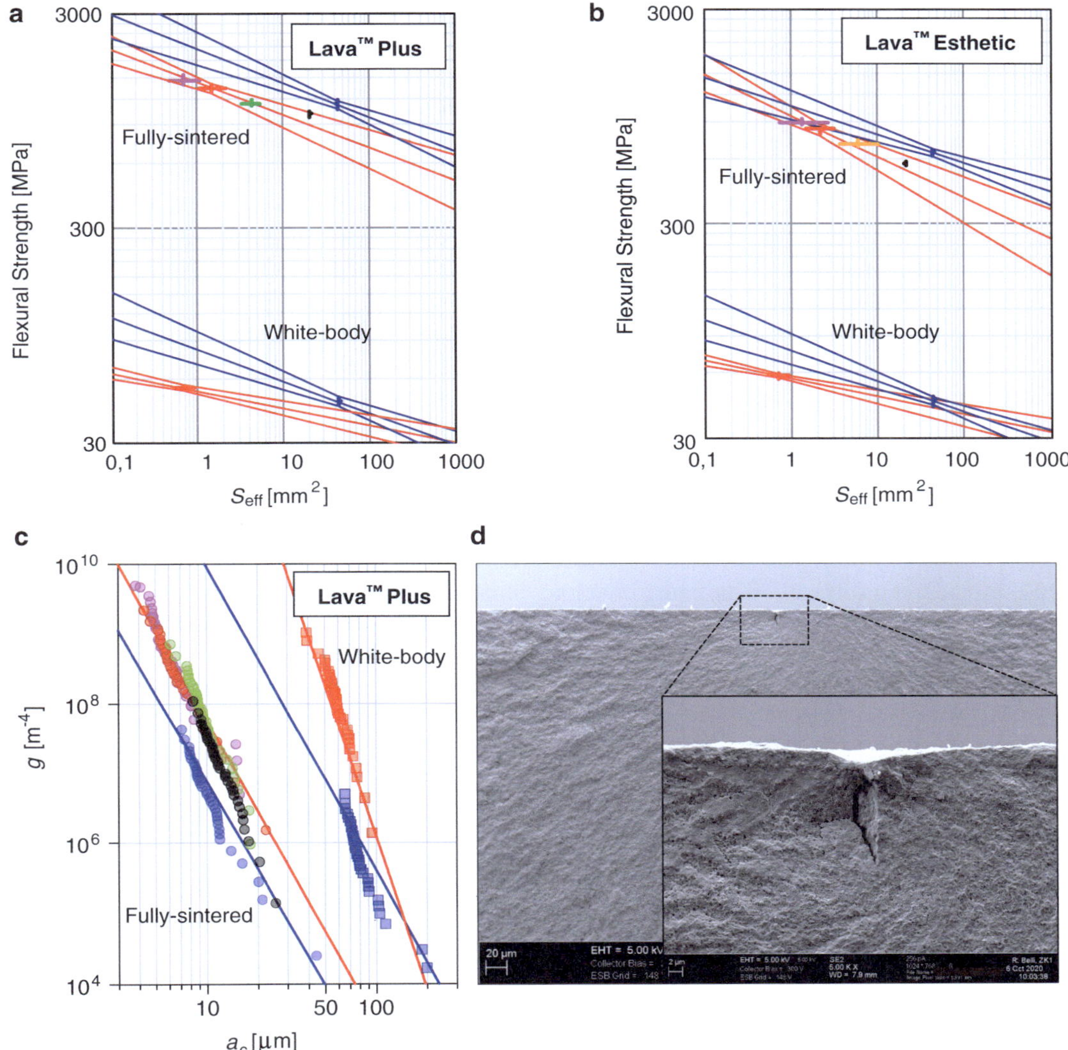

Fig. 2.17 Flexural strength vs. effective surfaces (S_{eff}) for the fully sintered and white bodies of a 3Y-TZP in (**a**) and for a 5Y-TZP in (**b**) for different specimen sizes, showing the deviation of the Weibull prediction for the largest specimen size. (**c**) shows lower values for the relative frequency flaw size density function $g(a)$ for the largest specimen, with its critical crack size a_{c} shifted to lower values. (**d**) shows a typical compaction defect (star) with a similar shape as in Fig. 2.16 being the critical defect triggering fracture in fully sintered specimens. From Ref. [100]. Reprinted with permission from Wiley

very similar across different powder manufacturers.

A consequence of the strength distribution being governed by compaction defects is that the size distribution of critical defect sizes must be related to the size distribution of granulates within the powders, and an upper threshold must therefore exist. This was suggested by Ref. [100] as the cause for all materials in Table 2.4 in failing to show a behavior befitting the size effect on strength, a requirement for materials to be considered Weibull materials. This is shown exemplarily for a 3Y-TZP and a 5Y-TZP in Fig. 2.17, where the red and blue predictions, based respectively on the strength of a small and the largest specimens, do not align was per a typical Weibull behavior. The largest specimen shows a shift toward higher strengths, suggesting that size distribution of compaction defects reached a plateau, with no other second defect distribution competing at this size scale. This also reveals that the applicability of zirconias for large volume constructs is benefited by this behavior, but the potential for smaller constructs is not entirely exhausted, provided that improvements in powder technology and compaction processes can be guided toward reducing junction gaps between granulates.

Sandblasting with alumina particles, a common procedure meant to increase the bonding potential of cements onto the intaglio zirconia surface, tends to increase the strength of 3Y-TZP [104] by inducing surface $t \rightarrow m$ transformation [89] with consequent generation of compressive stresses on the outer layer. If this layer is thick enough in the subsurface, compressive stresses may engulf existing surface defects and act as a shielding term similar to Eq. (2.8) [105].

2.3.5 Veneered-Zirconia Bilayers

Before any attempt to make zirconia more translucent for use as monolithic material, zirconia has been extensively used mostly as a thin infrastructure to be veneered with highly esthetic glass-rich porcelains. Some years in, the clinical application of veneered-zirconia took a blow in the form of reported high rates of chipping of the veneer material in clinical service [106–108]. That inconveniency triggered a wave of scientific interest targeting the causes of that increased susceptibility to fracture. Theoretical models and experimental observations gave insights on an expected thermal incompatibility issue ensuing from the low thermal diffusivity of zirconia, which generates a high thermal gradient within the veneer layer [109]. Factors such as the magnitude of the mismatch in linear coefficient of thermal expansion between both materials, the cooling rate employed through the glass transition temperature of the veneer, and the thickness

ratio zirconia:veneer were identified as contributing to the severity in the built-up of residual stresses in the veneer layer [110–114]. Laboratorial testing later confirmed those variables as playing decisive roles in determining the susceptibility of the veneer layer to fracture [115, 116]. Figure 2.18a shows, for example, increased lifetimes obtained for veneered-zirconia crowns that were cooled slowly inside the oven, compared with the protocol of bench cooling [117]. Evidences also negated any fault of the quality of the adhesion between layers [115, 118]; it was a chipping problem, not a delamination problem. Clinical recommendations from the scientific community advised using veneering materials with matching CTEs, performing slow-cooling protocols, and modelling so-called "anatomical copings" that allowed for a veneer layer having a more homogeneous thickness (see Fig. 2.18b). That reputational crisis helped in boosting the popularity of the monolithic use of zirconia, thus avoiding the veneer layer altogether.

2.3.6 Low-Temperature Degradation

Perhaps more famous than zirconia itself, is the term *Low-Temperature Degradation* (LTD), stemming from a spontaneous $t \rightarrow m$ transformation in the absence of any triggering mechanical stress, at temperatures as low as body temperature, sufficing the presence of moisture. Some use the alternative terminology *Hydrothermal Aging* for the same phenomenon. The exact underlying mechanism being nevertheless unresolved, some consensus is enjoyed by the theory that oxygen anions dissociated from water molecules destabilize the tetragonal symmetry by occupying the oxygen vacancies formerly created by the stabilizing oxide (in this case Y_2O_3) [119]. This process begins at the surface with grain uplifting and roughening and progresses to the subsurface following a diffusion-controlled nucleation-and-growth process [120], with the stress induced by the volume increase setting off the transformation of neighboring grains. As the transformed zone evolves inward into the bulk

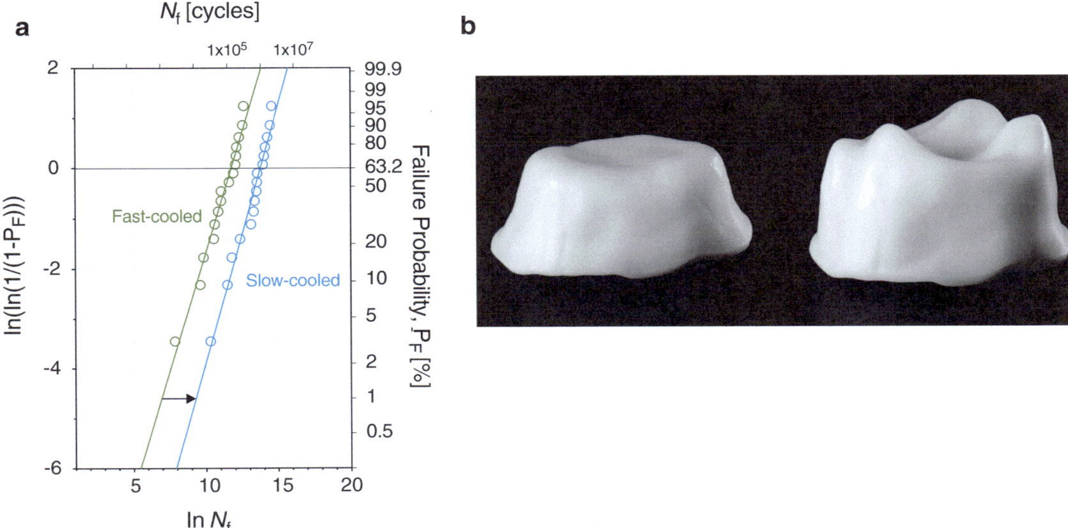

Fig. 2.18 (**a**) Weibull plot showing the lifetime of veneered-zirconia crowns having a high CTE mismatch and cooled down fast (bench cooling) or slow (under T_g inside the oven) loaded cyclically in a chewing simulator. (**b**) Conventional zirconia coping having a homogeneous thickness (left-hand side) and an "anatomically-shaped" coping (right-hand side)

material, microcracking, grain pull-out, and ultimately surface pitting mark the repercussions to the structural integrity. Due to signs of LTD being present throughout the surface and subsurface of recovered 3Y-TZPs belonging to a batch of femoral heads that had fractured clinically at an abnormally rapid rate in the early 2000s, LTD came into the spotlight as a potential vulnerability staining the great expectations for zirconia as a mechanically stable biomedical ceramic. Reverberations were felt across medical and engineering disciplines, reaching also dentistry, with the research community eager to find out to which degree were dental zirconias susceptible to any loss in expected performance. That episode of mass fracture of orthopedic 3Y-TZP hip implants was found to be due to newly introduced—deficient—fabrication steps leading to high porosity batches [121]. Subsequent machining of the sintered pieces had induced surface residual stresses, which is believed to have ignited a process (LTD) that usually takes a long time in the body to become significant.

Some mechanical testing have shown contradictory results; while negative effects of LTD on bending strength have been reported [122, 123], opposite results can also be found [124–126]. The effects of LTD on the strength are related to the layer of compressive (strengthening) stresses generated by the transformation, the compensating tensile (weakening) stress zone neighboring the transformed zone [127], and how this change in stress state affects the natural defect population of the material. For example, critical defects can be completely or only partly engulfed in this transformation layer, depending on their size distribution. Possibly, a different flaw population underneath of the transformation zone can become activated, thus starting to dominate the fracture initiation behavior [122]. Also, with the evolution of transformation toward the bulk, inter- and intragranular cracks start to develop within the transformed layer, in an orientation plane parallel to that of the surface. That particular orientation is less dangerous under bending conditions than if orthogonal to the surface, but if they coalesce, the transformed layer thickness can become itself the critical defect size. In other loading orientations composed of shear components, such as when contact wear is involved,

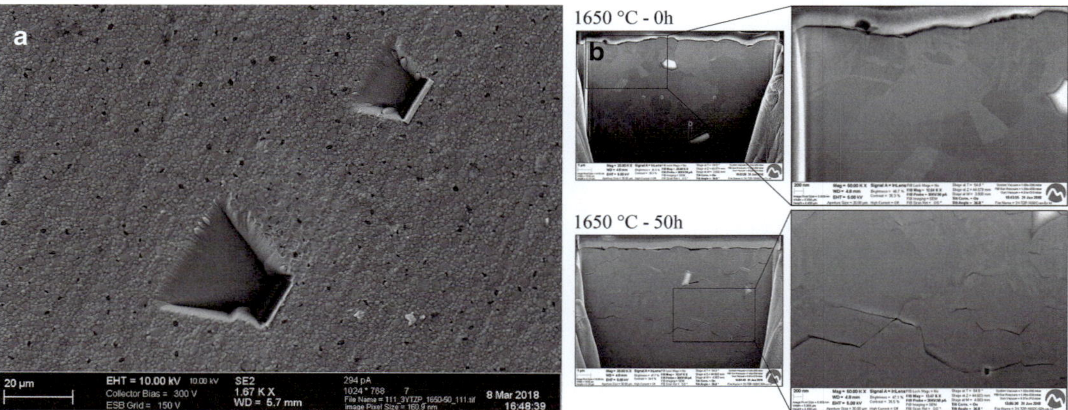

Fig. 2.19 (**a**) Surface of a 3Y-TZP material severely affected by LTD, with black spots being grain pull-outs. Focus-ion beam trenches are seen prepared on the surface for the evaluation of the subsurface material. (**b**) View from the prepared trenches of a 3Y-TZP sintered at 1650 °C after 0 or 50 h of accelerated aging in an autoclave at 134 °C. The pattern of transformation is already visible at the surface layer at 0 h, and extends 25 μm deep after 50 h, with severe cracks that develop in a plane parallel to the surface

those cracks can quickly become detrimental. In Fig. 2.19, the subsurface transformation zone is exposed by Focus-Ion Beam milling on a 3Y-TZP sintered at 1650 °C showing already one-grain-thick surface transformation due to larger grain sizes, and after 50 h of artificial aging, where extensive subsurface cracking is seen. Such effects are obviously dependent on how LTD is let on to evolve [123].

Many factors seem to affect the susceptibility to, and evolution rate of LTD, especially those compositions containing large amounts of the transformable *t*-phase; translucent zirconias are much less affected. Regarding 3Y-TZP, grain size (controlled mainly by sintering temperature) [128–130], amount of alloying oxides (Y_2O_3, CeO_2, Al_2O_3) [131–134], and initial amount of cubic phase [119] are most important factors. In dental implants, the most relevant are those concerning surface modification. Post-sintering sandblasting and roughening the surface, for example, have been shown to induce compressive stresses beneficial to the strength of the piece, increasing its resistance to LTD [135, 136], while annealing promotes the reverse effect [135].

Although LTD is referred to as a malignant process that is expected to lead to mechanical degradation [126, 137], especially when wear is involved, its clinical relevance is yet to be defined on the framework of a clinical setting. To date, there are still no clinical trials singling out LTD as either main or contributing cause to clinical failure in dental prosthetic constructs. Laboratorial experiments seem to negate such a pessimistic view of LTD as an agent that limits the lifetime of 3Y-TZP, providing even indication of an increase in fatigue resistance [126, 138–140].

2.4 Hybrid Ceramics

The subset of hybrid ceramics holds an important place in the historical development of all-ceramic systems for dentistry, allowing in the 1990s reinforced infrastructures for bridges to be constructed without metallic components for the first time. The first hybrid ceramics consisted of three variants according to the composition of the polycrystalline scaffold: Al_2O_3, Al_2O_3 + Ce-ZrO_2, and $MgAl_2O_4$, respectively, InCeram® Alumina, InCeram® Zirconia, and InCeram® Spinell. The latter was slightly more translucent and used exclusively for the anterior region. The slip (dispersion of powder in water) was applied using the *slip-casting* technique directly on top of the plaster dye abutment and formed by hand, subsequently undergoing a partial sintering firing. That firing took place at lower temperatures (~1100 °C) than the sintering temperature necessary to fully sinter those materials, so that the polycrystalline particles would only partially fuse together and an interconnecting porosity would remain. In a second step, a Lanthanum oxide-rich glass slip was applied by hand on top of the partially sintered polycrystalline scaffold, which infiltrated the porosity during a second firing, ultimately providing cohesion to the piece. Lanthanum oxide was used to improve the thermal compatibility between the glass and the polycrystalline phases and improve the refractive index. These products were later on made available for machining, the so-called *dry-pressed* version. In InCeram® Alumina (~68 vol.% Al_2O_3, 28 vol.% glass, ~4 vol.% porosity), the dry pressed version showed a more equiaxial microstructural shape, resulting in lower fracture toughness (3.6 MPa√m) than the elongated particles in the slip-cast version (4.4 MPa√m) [141]. For InCeram® Zirconia (~34 vol.% Al_2O_3, ~34 vol.% ZrO_2, 22 vol.% glass, ~10 vol.% porosity) both versions showed a mixture of elongated and rounded granules, resulting in equivalent mechanical properties (both ~4.8 MPa√m) [142]; those values might be a bit overestimated due to the testing method employed using Vickers indentations. Compared to polycrystalline ceramics, both InCeram® Alumina and InCeram® Zirconia are more susceptible to grinding damage and strength degradation [143]. The high amount of glass and porosity in these systems still consisted of the weakest link [144], limiting their mechanical performance and application in longer span constructs. Due to the high opacity, laborious processing, and lower mechanical properties, the InCeram® Alumina and InCeram® Zirconia hybrid materials lost substantial ground during the 2000s to their direct competitors, namely polycrystalline zirconia and polycrystalline alumina, being thus discontinued for commercialization by the manufacturer in 2015.

The manufacturer of the hybrid InCeram® materials, i.e., Vita Zahnfabrik, employed a similar synthesis approach to fabricate a glass–polymer hybrid material for CAD-CAM processing branded Enamic®, having Young's modulus of ~37 GPa—in the intermediary range between conventional resin composites and glassy ceramics, thus aimed for competing in both markets. The inorganic phase is constituted of an aluminosilicate glass powder compact containing low fractions of crystalline particulates of some tectosilicate sort and trace amounts of baddeleyite [24]. The ceramic network structure is formed by irregular-shaped particulates having approx. 1–10 µm in size, interrupted at the beginning of the stage of neck formation by partial sintering with necks of approx. 0.1–2 µm in cross-section, resulting in an open concave pore geometry. The internal ceramic surface is treated with a silane coupling agent in order to increase wetting and provide chemical bonding to the subsequent monomer mixture. That mixture is composed of urethane dimethacrylate (UDMA) and triethylene glycol dimethacrylate (TEGDMA) with sufficiently low viscosity for infiltration, with curing taking place under high pressure to reduce shrinkage effects [145]. The final material contains ~75 vol.% ceramic phase and a ~ 25 vol.% polymer fraction. The microstructure of Enamic® is shown in Fig. 2.20.

Although promised to confer improved mechanical performance and indicated by the manufacturer for constructs as thin as 1 mm, the structure of Enamic® has been shown not to necessarily upgrade the performance of the materials

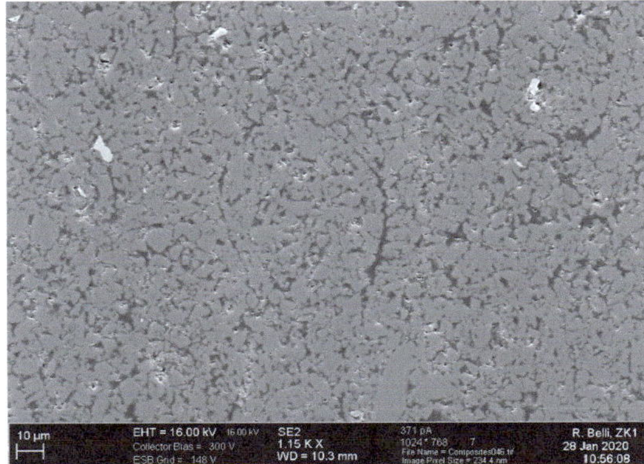

Fig. 2.20 SEM image of the microstructure of Enamic®, showing the glassy scaffold (lighter phase) and the infiltrated polymer (darker phase). From Ref. [146]. Reprinted with permission from Elsevier

it tries to distinguish itself from (resin composites). In terms of wear and contact fatigue [147], as well as flexural strength [43], fracture toughness ($\sim$1.12 MPa$\sqrt{\text{m}}$) [4, 148, 149], edge strength [150], and marginal strength [151], Enamic® performed similarly or worse than conventional resin composites. Additionally, the claim of Enamic® presenting an *R-curve* behavior [145, 152, 153] has not been corroborated [4, 146]. Despite the hype involving infiltrated scaffold materials, there is little basis for justifying their use instead of conventional resin composites and/or glass-ceramics, seen from a mechanical standpoint.

References

1. Thompson LM, Stebbins JF. Non-bridging oxygen and high-coordinated aluminum in meta- luminous and peraluminous calcium and potassium aluminosilicate glasses: high-resolution 17O and 27Al MAS NMR results. Am Mineral Am Mineral. 2011;96:841–53.
2. Quinn JB, Sundar V, Lloyd IK. Influence of microstructure and chemistry on the fracture toughness of dental ceramics. Dent Mater. 2003;19:603–11.
3. Scherrer SS, Kelly JR, Quinn GD, Xu K. Fracture toughness (K-Ic) of a dental porcelain determined by fractographic analysis. J Dent Res. 1998;77:656.
4. Belli R, Wendler M, Petschelt A, Lube T, Lohbauer U. Fracture toughness testing of biomedical ceramic-based materials using beams, plates and discs. J Eur Ceram Soc. 2018;38:5533–44.
5. Mackert JR Jr, Butts MB, Fairhurst CW. The effect of the leucite transformation on dental porcelain expansion. Dent Mater. 1986;2:32–6.
6. Zhang Y, Rao PG, Lu M, Wu JQ. Mechanical properties of dental porcelain with different leucite particle sizes. J Am Ceram Soc. 2008;91:527–34.
7. Zhang Y, Qu C, Rao PG, Lu MC, Wu JQ. Nanocrystalline seeding effect on the crystallization of two leucite precusors. J Am Ceram Soc. 2007;90:2390–8.
8. Cattell MJ, Patzig C, Bissasu S, Tsoutsos A, Karpukhina N. Nucleation efficacy and flexural strength of novel leucite glass-ceramics. Dent Mater. 2020;36:592–602.
9. Denry IL, Mackert JR Jr, Holloway JA, Rosenstiel SF. Effect of cubic leucite stabilization on the flexural strength of feldspathic dental porcelain. J Dent Res. 1996;75:1928–35.
10. Cesar PF, Yoshimura HN, Miranda Junior WG, Okada CY. Correlation between fracture toughness and leucite content in dental porcelains. J Dent. 2005;33:721–9.
11. Lee HH, Kon M, Asaoka K. Influence of modification of Na2O in a glass matrix on the strength of leucite-containing porcelains. Dent Mater J. 1997;16:134–43.
12. Kon M, Kawano F, Asaoka K, Matsumoto N. Effect of leucite crystals on the strength of glassy porcelain. Dent Mater J. 1994;13:138–47.
13. Belli R, Petschelt A, Hofner B, Hajto J, Scherrer SS, Lohbauer U. Fracture rates and lifetime estimations of CAD/CAM all-ceramic restorations. J Dent Res. 2016;95:67–73.
14. Belli R, Wendler M, Cicconi MR, de Ligny D, Petschelt A, Werbach K, et al. Fracture anisotropy in texturized lithium disilicate glass-ceramics. J Non-Cryst Solids. 2018;481:457–69.
15. Huang SF, Li Y, Wei SH, Huang ZH, Gao W, Cao P. A novel high-strength lithium disilicate glass-ceramic featuring a highly intertwined microstructure. J Eur Ceram Soc. 2017;37:1083–94.
16. Zanotto ED. A bright future for glass-ceramics. Am Ceram Soc Bull. 2010;89:19–27.
17. Beall GH. Dr. S. Donald (Don) Stookey (1915-2014): pioneering researcher and adventurer. Front Mater. 2016;3:37.
18. Lubauer J, Belli R, Peterlik H, Hurle K, Lohbauer U. Grasping the lithium hype: insights into modern lithium silicate glass-ceramics. Dental Mater. 2021;38(2):318–32.
19. Soares PC, Zanotto ED, Fokin VM, Jain H. TEM and XRD study of early crystallization of lithium disilicate glasses. J Non-Cryst Solids. 2003;331:217–27.
20. Gaddam A, Fernandes HR, Tulyaganov DU, Ribeiro MJ, Ferreira JMF. The roles of P2O5 and SiO2/Li2O ratio on the network structure and crystallization kinetics of non-stoichiometric lithium disilicate based glasses. J Non-Cryst Solids. 2018;481:512–21.
21. Ortiz AL, Rodrigues CS, Guiberteau F, Zhang Y. An in situ and ex situ study of the microstructural evolution of a novel lithium silicate glass-ceramic during crystallization firing. Dent Mater. 2020;36:645–59.
22. Lubauer J, Hurle K, Cicconi MR, Petschelt A, Peterlik H, Lohbauer U. Toughening by revitrification of Li2SiO3 crystals in Obsidian dental glass-ceramic. J Mech Behav Biomed Mater. 2021;124:104739.
23. Hurle K, Belli R, Götz-Neunhoeffer F, Lohbauer U. Phase characterization of lithium silicate biomedical glass-ceramics produced by two-stage crystallization. J Non-Cryst Solids. 2019;510:42–50.
24. Belli R, Wendler M, de Ligny D, Cicconi MR, Petschelt A, Peterlik H, et al. Chairside CAD/CAM materials. Part 1: measurement of elastic constants and microstructural characterization. Dent Mater. 2017;33:84–98.
25. Lin CC, Shen PY, Chang HM, Yang YJ. Composition dependent structure and elasticity of lithium silicate glasses: effect of ZrO2 additive and the combi-

nation of alkali silicate glasses. J Eur Ceram Soc. 2006;26:3613–20.

26. Kruger S, Deubener J, Ritzberger C, Holand W. Nucleation kinetics of lithium metasilicate in ZrO2-bearing lithium Disilicate glasses for dental application. Int J Appl Glas Sci. 2013;4:9–19.

27. Thieme K, Russel C. Nucleation and growth kinetics and phase analysis in zirconia-containing lithium disilicate glass. J Mater Sci. 2015;50:1488–99.

28. Matusita K, Sakka S, Maki T, Tashiro M. Study on crystallization of glass by differential thermal-analysis—effect of added oxide on crystallization of Li2o-Sio2 glasses. J Mater Sci. 1975;10:94–100.

29. Fernandes HR, Tulyaganov DU, Ferreira JMF. The role of P2O5, TiO2 and ZrO2 as nucleating agents on microstructure and crystallization behaviour of lithium disilicate-based glass. J Mater Sci. 2013;48:765–73.

30. Apel E, van't Hoen C, Rheinberger V, Holand W. Influence of ZrO2 on the crystallization and properties of lithium disilicate glass-ceramics derived from a multi-component system. J Eur Ceram Soc. 2007;27:1571–7.

31. Huang X, Zheng X, Zhao G, Zhong B, Zhang X, Wen G. Microstructure and mechanical properties of zirconia-toughened lithium disilicate glass-ceramic composites. Mater Chem Phys. 2014;143:845–52.

32. Zanotto ED, Leite MLG. The nucleation mechanism of lithium disilicate glass revisited. J Non-Cryst. Solids 1996;202:145–52.

33. Iqbal Y, Lee WE, Holland D, James PF. Metastable phase formation in the early stage crystallisation of lithium disilicate glass. J Non-Cryst Solids. 1998;224:1–16.

34. Zanotto ED. Metastable phases in lithium disilicate glasses. J Non-Cryst Solids. 1997;219:42–8.

35. Deubener J, Bruckner R, Sternitzke M. Induction time analysis of nucleation and crystal-growth in disilicate and metasilicate glasses. J Non-Cryst Solids. 1993;163:1–12.

36. Huang SF, Huang ZH, Gao W, Cao P. Structural response of lithium disilicate in glass crystallization. Cryst Growth Des. 2014;14:5144–51.

37. Bischoff C, Eckert H, Apel E, Rheinberger VM, Holand W. Phase evolution in lithium disilicate glass-ceramics based on non-stoichiometric compositions of a multi-component system: structural studies by Si-29 single and double resonance solid state NMR. Phys Chem Chem Phys. 2011;13:4540–51.

38. Hesse KF. Refinement of the crystal structure of lithium polysilicate. Acta Crystallogr. 1977;B33:901–2.

39. De Jong BHWS, Super HTJ, Spek AL, Veldman N, Nachtegaal G, Fischer JC. Mixed alkali systems: structure and Si-29 MASNMR of Li2Si2O5 and K2Si2O5. Acta Crystallogr B. 1998;54:568–77.

40. Momma K, Izumi F. VESTA 3 for three-dimensional visualization of crystal, volumetric and morphology data. J Appl Crystallogr. 2011;44:1272–6.

41. Lubauer J, Belli R, Petschelt A, Cicconi MR, Hurle K, Lohbauer U. Concurrent kinetics of crystallization and toughening in multicomponent biomedical SiO2-Li2O-P2O5-ZrO2 glass-ceramics. J Non-Cryst Solids. 2021;554:120607.

42. Belli R, Lohbauer U, Goetz-Neunhoeffer F, Hurle K. Crack-healing during two-stage crystallization of biomedical lithium (di)silicate glass-ceramics. Dent Mater. 2019;35:1130–45.

43. Wendler M, Belli R, Petschelt A, Mevec D, Harrer W, Lube T, et al. Chairside CAD/CAM materials. Part 2: flexural strength testing. Dent Mater. 2017;33:99–109.

44. Santos GG, Serbena FC, Fokin VM, Zanotto ED. Microstructure and mechanical properties of nucleant-free Li2O-CaO-SiO2 glass-ceramics. Acta Mater. 2017;130:347–60.

45. Mastelaro VR, Zanotto ED. Anisotropic residual stresses in partially crystallized Li2=-2SiO2 glass-ceramics. J Non-Cryst Solids. 1999;247:79–86.

46. Villas-Boas MOC, Serbena FC, Soares VO, Mathias I, Zanotto ED. Residual stress effect on the fracture toughness of lithium disilicate glass-ceramics. J Am Ceram Soc. 2020;103:465–79.

47. Oh W-S, Zhang N-Z, Anusavice KJ. Effect of heat treatment on fracture toughness (KIc) and microstructure of a fluorcanasite-based glass-ceramic. J Prosthodont. 2007;16:439–44.

48. Yoshimura HN, Cesar PF, Miranda WG, Gonzaga CC, Okada CY, Goldenstein H. Fracture toughness of dental porcelains evaluated by IF, SCF, and SEPB methods. J Am Ceram Soc. 2005;88:1680–3.

49. Serbena FC, Mathias I, Foester CE, Zanotto ED. Crystallization toughening of a model glass-ceramic. Acta Mater. 2015;86:216–28.

50. Belli R, Wendler M, Zorzin JI, Lohbauer U. Practical and theoretical considerations on the fracture toughness testing of dental restorative materials. Dent Mater. 2018;34:97–119.

51. Quinn GD, Swab JJ, Patel P. Fracture toughness of modern and ancient glasses and glass ceramics as measured by the SEPB method. Ceram Eng Sci Proc. 2018;39:1–11.

52. Soares VO, Serbena FC, Mathias I, Crovace MC, Zanotto ED. New, tough and strong lithium metasilicate dental glass-ceramic. Ceramics International. 2020;47(2):2793–801.

53. Kirsten J, Belli R, Wendler M, Petschelt A, Hurle K, Lohbauer U. Crack growth rates in lithium disilicates with bulk (mis)alignment of the Li2Si2O5 phase in the [001] direction. J Non-Cryst Solids. 2020;532:119877.

54. Gonzaga CC, Okada CY, Cesar PF, Miranda WG Jr, Yoshimura HN. Effect of processing induced particle alignment on the fracture toughness and fracture behavior of multiphase dental ceramics. Dent Mater. 2009;25:1293–301.

55. Albakry M, Guazzato M, Swain MV. Influence of hot-pressing on the microstructure and fracture toughness of two pressable dental glass-ceramics. J Biomed Mater Res B Appl Biomater. 2004;71B:99–107.

56. Belli R, Wendler M, Petschelt A, Lohbauer U. Mixed-mode fracture toughness of texturized LS2 glass-ceramics using the three-point bending with eccentric notch test. Dent Mater. 2017;33:1473–7.

57. Belli R, Wendler W, Zorzin JI, da Silva LH, Petschelt A, Lohbauer U. Fracture toughness mode mixity at the connectors of monolithic 3Y.TZP and LS2 dental bridge constructs. J Eur Ceram Soc. 2015;35:3701–11.

58. Curran P, Cattani-Lorente M, Wiskott HWA, Durual S, Scherrer SS. Grinding damage assessment for CAD-CAM restorative materials. Dent Mater. 2017;33:294–308.

59. Lohbauer U, Muller FA, Petschelt A. Influence of surface roughness on mechanical strength of resin composite versus glass ceramic materials. Dent Mater. 2008;24:250–6.

60. Belli R, Volkl H, Csato S, Tremmel S, Wartzack S, Lohbauer U. Development of a hoop-strength test for model sphero-cylindrical dental ceramic crowns: FEA and fractography. J Eur Ceram Soc. 2020;40:4753–64.

61. Tanaka S, Chia-Pin C, Kato Z, Uematsu K. Effect of internal binder on microstructure in compacts made from granules. J Eur Ceram Soc. 2007;27:873–7.

62. Tanaka S, Pin CC, Uematsu K. Effect of organic binder segregation on sintered strength of dry-pressed alumina. J Am Ceram Soc. 2006;89:1903–7.

63. Zhang Y, Suga T, Kawasaki M, Tang XX, Uchida N, Uematsu K. Effect of poly(vinyl alcohol) adsorption on binder segregation during drying. J Am Ceram Soc. 1996;79:435–40.

64. Hondo T, Yasuda K, Wakai F, Tanaka S. Influence of binder layer of spray-dried granules on occurrence and evolution of coarse defects in alumina ceramics during sintering. J Eur Ceram Soc. 2018;38:1846–52.

65. Kelly JR, Denry I. Stabilized zirconia as a structural ceramic: an overview. Dent Mater. 2008;24:289–98.

66. Denry I, Kelly JR. State of the art of zirconia for dental applications. Dent Mater. 2008;24:299–307.

67. Li P, Chen IW. Effect of dopants on zirconia stabilization—an X-Ray-absorption study. 2. Tetravalent dopants. J Am Ceram Soc. 1994;77:1281–8.

68. Li P, Chen IW, Pennerhahn JE. Effect of dopants on zirconia stabilization—an X-ray-absorption study. 1. Trivalent dopants. J Am Ceram Soc. 1994;77:118–28.

69. Guo X. Property degradation of tetragonal zirconia induced by low-temperature defect reaction with water molecules. Chem Mater. 2004;16:3988–94.

70. Fabris S, Paxton AT, Finnis MW. A stabilization mechanism of zirconia based on oxygen vacancies only. Acta Mater. 2002;50:5171–8.

71. Kawata K, Maekawa H, Nemoto T, Yamamura T. Local structure analysis of YSZ by Y-89 MAS-NMR. Solid State Ionics. 2006;177:1687–90.

72. Fabrichnaya O, Aldinger F. Assessment of thermodynamic parameters in the system ZrO2-Y2O3-Al2O3. Z Metallkunde. 2004;95:27–39.

73. Lakiza S, Fabrichnaya O, Zinkevich M, Aldinger F. On the phase relations in the ZrO2-YO1.5-AlO1.5 system. J Alloys Compd. 2006;420:237–45.

74. Kilo M, Taylor MA, Argirusis C, Borchardt G, Lesage B, Weber S, et al. Cation self-diffusion of ca-44, Y-88, and Zr-96 in single-crystalline calcia- and yttria-doped zirconia. J Appl Phys. 2003;94:7547–52.

75. Lanteri V, Chaim R, Heuer AH. On the microstructures resulting from the diffusionless cubic—tetragonal transformation in Zro2-Y2o3 alloys. J Am Ceram Soc. 1986;69:C258–C61.

76. Scott HG. Phase relationships in zirconia-Yttria system. J Mater Sci. 1975;10:1527–35.

77. Virkar AV, Matsumoto RLK. Ferroelastic domain switching as a toughening mechanism in tetragonal zirconia. J Am Ceram Soc. 1986;69:C224–C6.

78. Yashima M, Ishizawa N, Yoshimura M. High temperature x-ray diffraction study on cubic-tetragonal phase transition in the ZrO2-RO1.5 systems (R: rare earths). In: Badwal SPS, Bannister MJ, Hannink RHJ, editors. Science and Technology of Zirconia. Lancaster: Technomic; 1993. p. 125–35.

79. Krogstad JA, Lepple M, Gao Y, Lipkin DM, Levi CG. Effect of Yttria content on the zirconia unit cell parameters. J Am Ceram Soc. 2011;94:4548–55.

80. Krogstad JA, Kramer S, Lipkin DM, Johnson CA, Mitchell DRG, Cairney JM, et al. Phase stability of t′-zirconia-based thermal barrier coatings: mechanistic insights. J Am Ceram Soc. 2011;94:S168–S77.

81. Lipkin DM, Krogstad JA, Gao Y, Johnson CA, Nelson WA, Levi CG. Phase evolution upon aging of air-plasma sprayed t′-zirconia coatings: I-Synchrotron X-ray diffraction. J Am Ceram Soc. 2013;96:290–8.

82. Krogstad JA, Gao Y, Bai JM, Wang J, Lipkin DM, Levi CG. In situ diffraction study of the high-temperature decomposition of t′-zirconia. J Am Ceram Soc. 2015;98:247–54.

83. Inokoshi M, Shimizu H, Nozaki K, Takagaki T, Yoshihara K, Nagaoka N, et al. Crystallographic and morphological analysis of sandblasted highly translucent dental zirconia. Dent Mater. 2018;34:508–18.

84. Camposilvan E, Leone R, Gremillard L, Sorrentino R, Zarone F, Ferrari M, et al. Aging resistance, mechanical properties and translucency of different yttria-stabilized zirconia ceramics for monolithic dental crown applications. Dent Mater. 2018;34:879–90.

85. Kolakarnprasert N, Kaizer MR, Kim DK, Zhang Y. New multi-layered zirconias: composition, microstructure and translucency. Dent Mater. 2019;35:797–806.

86. Zhang F, Inokoshi M, Batuk M, Hadermann J, Naert I, Van Meerbeek B, et al. Strength, toughness and aging stability of highly-translucent Y-TZP ceramics for dental restorations. Dent Mater. 2016;32:e327–e37.

87. Krogstad JA, Leckie RM, Kramer S, Cairney JM, Lipkin DM, Johnson CA, et al. Phase evolution upon aging of air plasma sprayed t′-zirconia coatings: II-microstructure evolution. J Am Ceram Soc. 2013;96:299–307.

88. Belli R, Hurle K, Schürrlein J, Petschelt A, Werbach K, Peterlik H, et al. Relationships between fracture toughness, Y2O3 fraction and phases content in modern Yttria-doped zirconias. J Eur Ceram Soc. 2021;41(15):771–7782.

89. Grigore A, Spallek S, Petschelt A, Butz B, Spiecker E, Lohbauer U. Microstructure of veneered zirconia after surface treatments: a TEM study. Dent Mater. 2013;29:1098–107.

90. Zhang F, Reveron H, Spies BC, Van Meerbeek B, Chevalier J. Trade-off between fracture resistance and translucency of zirconia and lithium-disilicate glass ceramics for monolithic restorations. Acta Biomater. 2019;91:24–34.

91. Lange FF. Transformation Toughening. 3. Experimental-observations in the Zro2-Y2o3 system. J Mater Sci. 1982;17:240–6.

92. Zhang Y. Making yttria-stabilized tetragonal zirconia translucent. Dent Mater. 2014;30:1195–203.

93. Hannink RHJ, Kelly PM, Muddle BC. Transformation toughening in zirconia-containing ceramics. J Am Ceram Soc. 2000;83:461–87.

94. Kailer A, Stephan M. On the feasibility of the Chevron Notch Beam method to measure fracture toughness of fine-grained zirconia ceramics. Dent Mater. 2016;32:1256–62.

95. Miyazaki H, Yoshizawa Y. A reinvestigation of the validity of the indentation fracture (IF) method as applied to ceramics. J Eur Ceram Soc. 2017;37:4437–41.

96. Mercer C, Williams JR, Clarke DR, Evans AG. On a ferroelastic mechanism governing the toughness of metastable tetragonal-prime (t′) yttria-stabilized zirconia. Proc R Soc A. 2007;463:1393–408.

97. Basu B, Vleugels J, Van der Biest O. Toughness tailoring of yttria-doped zirconia ceramics. Mater Sci Eng A. 2004;380:215–21.

98. Smirnov A, Kurland HD, Grabow J, Muller FA, Bartolome JF. Microstructure, mechanical properties and low temperature degradation resistance of 2Y-TZP ceramic materials derived from nanopowders prepared by laser vaporization. J Eur Ceram Soc. 2015;35:2685–91.

99. Chevalier J, Taddei P, Gremillard L, Deville S, Fantozzi G, Bartolome JF, et al. Reliability assessment in advanced nanocomposite materials for orthopaedic applications. J Mech Behav Biomed Mater. 2011;4:303–14.

100. Belli R, Lohbauer U. The breakdown of the Weibull behavior in dental zirconias. J Am Ceram Soc. 2021;104(9):4819–28.

101. Scherrer SS, Cattani-Lorente M, Yoon S, Karvonen L, Pokrant S, Rothbrust F, et al. Post-hot isostatic pressing: a healing treatment for process related defects and laboratory grinding damage of dental zirconia? Dent Mater. 2013;29:E180–E90.

102. Scherrer S, Cesar PF, Lohbauer U, Belli R. Zirconia as a biomaterial in implant dentistry. Forum Implantol. 2018;14:6–17.

103. Boursier A, d'Esdra GG, Lintingre E, Fretigny C, Lequeux F, Talini L. Cold compression of ceramic spray-dried granules: role of the spatial distribution of the binder. Ceram Int. 2020;46:9680–90.

104. Inokoshi M, Shimizubata M, Nozaki K, Takagaki T, Yoshihara K, Minakuchi S, et al. Impact of sand-blasting on the flexural strength of highly translucent zirconia. J Mech Behav Biomed Mater. 2021;115:104268.

105. Caravaca CF, Flamant Q, Anglada M, Gremillard L, Chevalier J. Impact of sandblasting on the mechanical properties and aging resistance of alumina and zirconia based ceramics. J Eur Ceram Soc. 2018;38:915–25.

106. Sailer I, Pjetursson BE, Zwahlen M, Hammerle CHF. A systematic review of the survival and complication rates of all-ceramic and metal-ceramic reconstructions after an observation period of at least 3 years. Part II: fixed dental prostheses. Clin Oral Implan Res. 2007;18:86–96.

107. Sailer I, Feher A, Filser F, Gauckler LJ, Luthy H, Hammerle CHF. Five-year clinical results of zirconia frameworks for posterior fixed partial dentures. Int J Prosthodont. 2007;20:383–8.

108. Sailer I, Gottner J, Kanel S, Hammerle CHF. Randomized controlled clinical trial of zirconia-ceramic and metal-ceramic posterior fixed dental prostheses: a 3-year follow-up. Int J Prosthodont. 2009;22:553–60.

109. Swain MV. Unstable cracking (chipping) of veneering porcelain on all-ceramic dental crowns and fixed partial dentures. Acta Biomater. 2009;5:1668–77.

110. Belli R, Monteiro S, Baratieri LN, Katte H, Petschelt A, Lohbauer U. A Photoelastic assessment of residual stresses in zirconia-veneer crowns. J Dent Res. 2012;91:316–20.

111. Wendler M, Belli R, Petschelt A, Lohbauer U. Characterization of residual stresses in zirconia veneered bilayers assessed via sharp and blunt indentation. Dent Mater. 2015;31:948–57.

112. Choi JE, Waddell JN, Swain MV. Pressed ceramics onto zirconia. Part 2: indentation fracture and influence of cooling rate on residual stresses. Dent Mater. 2011;27:1111–8.

113. Wendler M, Belli R, Petschelt A, Lohbauer U. Spatial distribution of residual stresses in glass-ZrO2 sphero-cylindrical bilayers. J Mech Behav Biomed Mater. 2016;60:535–46.

114. Mainjot AK, Schajer GS, Vanheusden AJ, Sadoun MJ. Influence of cooling rate on residual stress profile in veneering ceramic: measurement by hole-drilling. Dent Mater. 2011;27:906–14.

115. Belli R, Petschelt A, Lohbauer U. Thermal-induced residual stresses affect the fractographic patterns of

zirconia-veneer dental prostheses. J Mech Behav Biomed Mater. 2013;21:167–77.

116. Mainjot AK, Schajer GS, Vanheusden AJ, Sadoun MJ. Residual stress measurement in veneering ceramic by hole-drilling. Dent Mater. 2011;27:439–44.

117. Belli R, Frankenberger R, Appelt A, Schmitt J, Baratieri LN, Greil P, et al. Thermal-induced residual stresses affect the lifetime of zirconia-veneer crowns. Dent Mater. 2013;29:181–90.

118. Tholey MJ, Swain MV, Thiel N. SEM observations of porcelain Y-TZP interface. Dent Mater. 2009;25:857–62.

119. Chevalier J, Gremillard L, Virkar AV, Clarke DR. The tetragonal-monoclinic transformation in zirconia: lessons learned and future trends. J Am Ceram Soc. 2009;92:1901–20.

120. Chevalier J, Cales B, Drouin JM. Low-temperature aging of Y-TZP ceramics. J Am Ceram Soc. 1999;82:2150–4.

121. Chevalier J, Gremillard L, Deville S. Low-temperature degradation of zirconia and implications for biomedical implants. Annu Rev Mater Res. 2007;37:1–32.

122. Marro FG, Mesta A, Anglada M. Weibull strength statistics of hydrothermally aged 3 Mol% yttria-stabilised tetragonal zirconia. Ceram Int. 2014;40:12777–82.

123. Siarampi E, Kontonasaki E, Andrikopoulos KS, Kantiranis N, Voyiatzis GA, Zorba T, et al. Effect of in vitro aging on the flexural strength and probability to fracture of Y-TZP zirconia ceramics for all-ceramic restorations. Dent Mater. 2014;30:E306–E16.

124. Kim HT, Han JS, Yang JH, Lee JB, Kim SH. The effect of low temperature on the mechanical property and phase stability of Y-TZP ceramics. J Adv Prosthodont. 2009;1:113–7.

125. Virkar AV, Huang JL, Cutler RA. Strengthening of oxide ceramics by transformation-induced stresses. J Am Ceram Soc. 1987;70:164–70.

126. Sanon C, Chevalier J, Douillard T, Kohal RJ, Coelho PG, Hjerppe J, et al. Low temperature degradation and reliability of one-piece ceramic oral implants with a porous surface. Dent Mater. 2013;29:389–97.

127. Caravaca CF, Flamant Q, Anglada M, Gremillard L, Chevalier J. Impact of sandblasting on the mechanical properties and aging resistance of alumina and zirconia based ceramics. J Eur Ceram Soc. 2018;38(3):15–925.

128. Li JF, Watanabe R. Phase transformation in Y2O3-partially-stabilized ZrO2 polycrystals of various grain sizes during low-temperature aging in water. J Am Ceram Soc. 1998;81:2687–91.

129. Cotic J, Jevnikar P, Kocjan A, Kosmac T. Complexity of the relationships between the sintering-temperature-dependent grain size, airborne-particle abrasion, ageing and strength of 3Y-TZP ceramics. Dent Mater. 2016;32:510–8.

130. Hallmann L, Mehl A, Ulmer P, Reusser E, Stadler J, Zenobi R, et al. The influence of grain size on low-temperature degradation of dental zirconia. J Biomed Mater Res B. 2012;100b:447–56.

131. Tsubakino H, Sonoda K, Nozato R. Martensite-transformation behavior during isothermal aging in partially-stabilized zirconia with and without alumina addition. J Mater Sci Lett. 1993;12:196–8.

132. Palmero P, Fornabaio M, Montanaro L, Reveron H, Esnouf C, Chevalier J. Towards long lasting zirconia-based composites for dental implants. Part I: innovative synthesis, microstructural characterization and in vitro stability. Biomaterials. 2015;50:38–46.

133. Zhang F, Vanmeensel K, Inokoshi M, Batuk M, Hadermann J, Van Meerbeek B, et al. 3Y-TZP ceramics with improved hydrothermal degradation resistance and fracture toughness. J Eur Ceram Soc. 2014;34:2453–63.

134. Hallmann L, Ulmer P, Reusser E, Louvel M, Hammerle CHF. Effect of dopants and sintering temperature on microstructure and low temperature degradation of dental Y-TZP-zirconia. J Eur Ceram Soc. 2012;32:4091–104.

135. Cattani-Lorente M, Scherrer SS, Durual S, Sanon C, Douillard T, Gremillard L, et al. Effect of different surface treatments on the hydrothermal degradation of a 3Y-TZP ceramic for dental implants. Dent Mater. 2014;30:1136–46.

136. Deville S, Chevalier J, Gremillard L. Influence of surface finish and residual stresses on the ageing sensitivity of biomedical grade zirconia. Biomaterials. 2006;27:2186–92.

137. Lughi V, Sergo V. Low temperature degradation -aging- of zirconia: a critical review of the relevant aspects in dentistry. Dent Mater. 2010;26:807–20.

138. Oblak C, Verdenik I, Swain MV, Kosmac T. Survival-rate analysis of surface treated dental zirconia (Y-TZP) ceramics. J Mater Sci. 2014;25:2255–64.

139. Kosmac T, Oblak C, Marion L. The effects of dental grinding and sandblasting on ageing and fatigue behavior of dental zirconia (Y-TZP) ceramics. J Eur Ceram Soc. 2008;28:1085–90.

140. Belli R, Loher C, Petschelt A, Cicconi MR, de Ligny D, Anglada M, et al. Low-temperature degradation increases the cyclic fatigue resistance of 3Y-TZP in bending. Dent Mater. 2020;36:1086–95.

141. Guazzato M, Albakry M, Ringer SP, Swain MV. Strength, fracture toughness and microstructure of a selection of all-ceramic materials. Part I. Pressable and alumina glass-infiltrated ceramics. Dent Mater. 2004;20:441–8.

142. Guazzato M, Albakry M, Ringer SP, Swain MV. Strength, fracture toughness and microstructure of a selection of all-ceramic materials. Part II. Zirconia-based dental ceramics. Dent Mater. 2004;20:449–56.

143. Canneto JJ, Cattani-Lorente M, Durual S, Wiskott AHW, Scherrer SS. Grinding damage assess-

ment on four high-strength ceramics. Dent Mater. 2016;32:171–82.

144. Lohbauer U, Petschelt A, Greil P. Lifetime prediction of CAD/CAM dental ceramics. J Biomed Mater Res. 2002;63:780–5.

145. Swain MV, Coldea A, Bilkhair A, Guess PC. Interpenetrating network ceramic-resin composite dental restorative materials. Dent Mater. 2016;32:34–42.

146. Belli R, Zorzin JI, Petschelt A, Lohbauer U, Rocca GT. Crack growth behavior of a biomedical polymer-ceramic interpenetrating scaffolds composite in the subcritical regimen. Eng Fract Mech. 2020;231:107014.

147. Wendler M, Kaizer MR, Belli R, Lohbauer U, Zhang Y. Sliding contact wear and subsurface damage of CAD/CAM materials against zirconia. Dental Mater. 2020;36:387–401.

148. Della Bona A, Corazza PH, Zhang Y. Characterization of a polymer-infiltrated ceramic-network material. Dent Mater. 2014;30:564–9.

149. Quinn GD, Swab JJ, Patel P. Fracture toughness of modern and ancient glasses and glass ceramics as measured by the SEPB method. Hoboken: Wiley; 2019.

150. Quinn GD. On edge chipping testing and some personal perspectives on the state of the art of mechanical testing. Dent Mater. 2015;31:26–36.

151. Lubauer J, Belli R, Schünemann FH, Matta RE, Wichmann M, Wartzack S, et al. Inner marginal strength of CAD/CAM materials is not affected by machining protocol. Biomater Invest Dent. 2021;8:119–28.

152. Coldea A, Fischer J, Swain MV, Thiel N. Damage tolerance of indirect restorative materials (including PICN) after simulated bur adjustments. Dent Mater. 2015;31:684–94.

153. Coldea A, Swain MV, Thiel N. In-vitro strength degradation of dental ceramics and novel PICN material by sharp indentation. J Mech Behav Biomed Mater. 2013;26:34–42.

The Mechanics of Fracture in Dental Ceramics

3

On August 14, 2018, a ~200-m section of the *Morandi bridge* in Genoa, Italy, a construction dated back to 1967, collapsed 45 m to the ground, killing 43 people. Although no definite reports exist as of this date, the two main factors believed to have been decisive in inducing failure, were: (1) *flawed design* and (2) *material degradation*. In the engineering vernacular, the term "design" refers to the geometry of the components responsible for carrying the load—such as the diameter of supporting cables, or the cross-sectional dimensions of the hanging elements. In turn, "degradation" of a material relates to processes involved in the loss of its structural integrity over time (decay, in a sense), when beset by sustained mechanical and chemical aggressions. Unfortunately, by the constitution of disasters, nothing in the case of the *Morandi bridge* points to virtues of exceptionality; it rather shares common causes with diverse accidents involving man-made structures, including airplane crashes, train derailments, building collapses, and many others. Not that natural materials are immune to degradation—in living organisms, this process is referred to as "*ageing.*" In civil and mechanical engineering, design issues can be dealt with by reshaping and/or overscaling parts. In prosthetic dentistry, design meets the constraints defined by anatomy. In all instances, degradation cannot be entirely circumvented.

Although mechanical failures get wide attention in bridge proportions, the underlying mechanisms of fracture are ubiquitous throughout several scales, be that of length or prominence. That is, those mechanisms responsible for structural damage in big things, act also in small things, for they start at the atomic level to grow visible at macroscopic dimensions. It holds therefore true, that the mechanical laws governing fracture of notable bridges also control, for instance, how ordinary dental restorations fail. Ultimately, in order to study the mechanical behavior of dental materials one cannot escape the scope of classical mechanics. The branch committed to this problem is called *fracture mechanics*.

A setting for the understanding of the mechanisms of fracture is provided by some fundamentals of composition and processing of ceramics for dentistry. To gain insights on how these materials come to fail, we adopt engineering procedures for the most part of this book, applying the basis of mechanical testing that is anchored in the principles of fracture mechanics. Some analytical approaches were used in the last chapter and can now accompany the technical utterance to better characterize the architecture of microstructural units and related mechanisms of crack growth. Structural–property relationships, as it turns out, set the stage for tolerance against damage, or for yield.

Although for the dental academic such approaches might appear rather abstract at first, ornamental at best, we provide thereby elementary descriptions of mechanical behaviors that are implicit in the everyday challenges of the oral environment. The properties we measure in units,

© The Author(s), under exclusive license to Springer Nature Switzerland AG 2022
U. Lohbauer, R. Belli, *Dental Ceramics*, https://doi.org/10.1007/978-3-030-94687-6_3

the effects we convey in plots, are active—behind the scenes—in the dental crown, in the dental implant, during chewing and clenching. The applicability of laboratorial testing is unmistakable. Debates on clinical relevance are trivial.

3.1   The Strength Concept

How much mechanical stress a material can sustain, induced by an applied external load, before catastrophic fracture ensues, is what the concept of "strength" is supposed to convey. Because stress scales up with the applied force, of course, strength becomes a measure that can be intuitively related to ranges of realistic service forces for a specific application. Biting forces are expected to be higher in posterior regions of the arch, thus materials used for substitution of molar teeth should show higher strength values than those used for premolars or anterior teeth. In fact, ISO 6872 [1] utilizes this rationale to issue recommendations that assign clinical indications according to the type of reconstruction (monolithic, infrastructure, crown, bridges, etc.) for increasing intervals of flexural strength.

There have been, however, admonitions against embracing the strength concept unrestrictedly as an unchangeable material property defining the ability of a material to resist fracture. Deviations from such a [fixed property-like] behavior in brittle materials (i.e., ceramics and glasses) were gained by a couple of observations: (1) that the strength values of a set of specimens seem to follow a particular probability function, and; (2) that the probability of failure increases with the size of the specimens. These are products of the underlying nature of fracture described in modern fracture mechanics, built upon the principle that failure originates from physical entities such as flaws and defects that act as stress concentrators. As will be seen in Sect. 3.2, the length of the flaw is of main importance here, so that the largest flaw with the most unfavorable orientation in the stress field, will be the one triggering fracture. Naturally, there will be no single defect of random size for each specimen within a set of specimens, but rather the sizes of the many defects in a material (or specimen) and within a

set of specimens follows that particular distribution function seen defining the distribution of strength [2]. Meaning that there is a correlation between the strength distribution and the flaw size distribution.

Today's most accepted and applied statistical model of brittle fracture was developed by W. Weibull based on the weakest link hypothesis, which implies that the material fails once its weakest volume unit fails, as opposed to many elements simultaneously or all at once [3, 4]. Weibull's failure probability function F is given for a uniaxial homogeneous tensile stress state σ, in specimens of volume V, having noninteracting flaws:

$$F(\sigma,V) = 1 - \exp\left[-\frac{V}{V_0}\left(\frac{\sigma}{\sigma_0}\right)^m\right] \quad (3.1)$$

with V_0 and σ_0 being the characteristic volume and strength values, respectively, which represent a probability of failure of 63.2% when $V = V_0$ and $\sigma = \sigma_0$. The exponent m is the Weibull modulus, and describes the scatter of the strength values. The scale (σ_0) and the shape (m) terms are the Weibull parameters, which are usually sufficient to describe the distribution of strength in the absence of a superposed heterogeneous stress field (such as when a residual stress layer is present). The Weibull parameters can be derived from a $\ln(\sigma)$ vs. $\ln\ln(1/(1 - F))$ plot, with an estimation function $F_i = (i - \frac{1}{2})/X$, with X being the total number of specimens in a set, and i their individual rankings of ascending strength values. As in any statistical procedure, the higher the X (range of failure probabilities that was actually measured), the lower is the uncertainty of extrapolation (the confidence bounds get narrower). Technical standards [5] require a minimum of 30 specimens, as a compromise between cost of specimen fabrication and statistical accuracy. Antithetical to that argument, the dental standard ISO 6872 requires a minimum of 15 specimens and only *recommends* that 30 specimens are measured. We recommend to stick with the guidelines of technical standards. A least-squares regression can be used to fit the data points, but a more accurate procedure, such as the Maximum Likelihood Estimation method, is preferred. The

Weibull modulus is the slope of that curve, and the characteristic strength is the projection of the $\ln\ln(1/(1 - F)) = 0$ (or $F = 0.632$) toward the *x*-axis. The calculation of the confidence intervals is described in Ref. [5], and a significant difference is usually assumed when the confidence bounds fail to overlap.

An example of two strength datasets in a Weibull plot representation is shown in Fig. 3.1. The blue material shows a higher scale (located more to the right-hand side) and shape (steeper slope) parameters. When the data aligns well onto the regression, it can be assumed that the data distribution fits well to a Weibull distribution, as seems to be the case for the blue dataset rather than for the purple dataset. The most frequent reason for deviations from a straight data trend is the existence of additional flaw populations within the same set of specimens, other than a predominant parent flaw population of the same nature. This can take place due to a second type (bimodal) of flaw appearing within a narrow size range within that tested volume (seen in Fig. 3.1 by the "bump" in the purple dataset between $F = 0.1$ and $F = 0.5$), or be due to other effects, such as residual compressive stresses or R-curve behavior [6]. One might therefore be compelled to perform additional fractographic analysis of the entire dataset in order to gain some insight on the types of defect contained therein, and to be able to identify secondary populations or "artificial" defects than pollute the flaw population one is seeking to evaluate, such as when fractures originate from edge defects or unwanted grinding damage.

Strength-limiting defects can be of different natures in dental ceramic materials, and, as in other ceramic materials, they cannot be disentangled from the fabrication process used. Pressable glass-ceramics, for instance, usually contain a large amount of pores and a rough surface topography due to contact with the investment material and subsequent sandblasting procedure. Veneered porcelains used to cover opaque infrastructures may develop thermal flaws between separately fired veneer layers, acting as a volume defect if the contact load becomes critical [7]. In turn, defects in dental zirconias stem from sintering voids related to the inability of the powder aggregate particles to be sufficiently compacted [8]. Fractures in CAD/CAM glass-ceramics are often surface cracks caused by CAM grinding, if not eliminated by polishing. Grinding for adjustment of the internal fit also have shown to trigger clinical fractures [9]. In two-step glass-ceramics that need a second heat treatment after machining, the smear-layer produced by grinding, if not properly removed, can partially melt on the surface and form a pore-rich layer that acts as fracture sites [10].

Other flaw types are not inherent of the material itself (e.g., inhomogeneities, porosity, and large grains), but are artificially introduced to the test specimen during preparation, like edge damage due to sawing and surface damage due to grinding procedures. There can be therefore a combination of natural and artificial defects within a set of specimens, should their size scales overlap. When surface defects are dominating the fracture behavior, the volume in Eq. (3.1) must be replaced by the surface S. For a combination of volume and surface flaws, Eq. (3.1) reads [11]:

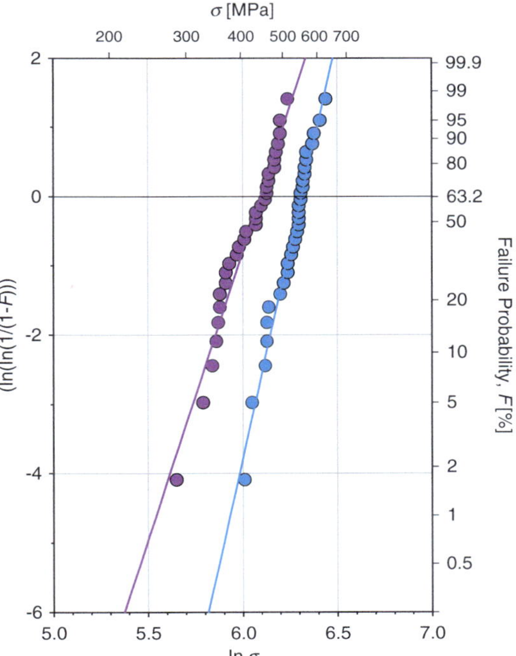

Fig. 3.1 Example of a Weibull plot containing two datasets of 30 specimens each. The blue material shows a higher characteristic strength and a higher Weibull modulus. The purple dataset does not seem to fit a Weibull distribution, possibly due to a second flaw population embedded in the parent flaw population

$$F(\sigma,V,S) = 1 - \exp\left[-\frac{V}{V_0}\left(\frac{\sigma_V}{\sigma_{V,0}}\right)^{m_V} - \frac{S}{S_0}\left(\frac{\sigma_S}{\sigma_{S,0}}\right)^{m_S}\right],\qquad(3.2)$$

and the Weibull plot will be formed by a slope at the lower strength tail transitioning into a slope dominating the upper tail of the strength distribution. The modelling of multiple flaw populations within the Weibull distribution function for the same volume or surface can be done similarly.

In mostly amorphous materials, which contain no microstructure that can act as defects, such as glasses, fracture originates mainly on the surface once the material becomes sensitive to very small crack sizes; even the most diligent polishing protocols may leave scratches that will be the triggering defects. In dental ceramics, one should therefore have the purpose of strength testing well thought out in advance: is the distribution of the natural occurring flaws, or rather relevant handling effects, to be evaluated? That will help define the specimen fabrication and preparation protocol, particularly concerning the surface quality. It might be insightful, for example, to machine specimens of CAD/CAM materials directly in the machining unit in order to determine a clinically relevant worst-case scenario. These will probably mask inherent (smaller) material-related defects, and will not contribute to exposing possible measures that can be undertaken for material improvement. If polishing is conducted on machined specimens, clinical polishing protocols would maintain the aspect of clinical relevance intact, as opposed to using laboratorial polishing equipment.

3.1.1   The Size Effect on Strength

There is considerable controversy on whether using Weibull statistics for treating strength datasets of ceramic materials is at all appropriate, instead of resorting to more simple statistical treatments assuming other types of distribution (e.g. normal and log-normal). Although very large datasets have established

that some ceramic materials do fit a Weibull distribution better [12], commonly tested sample sizes under standard recommendations have been shown to be insufficient for differences between similar distributions to be distinguished [13]. Thus, one is at most assuming that it is being dealt with a Weibull material. That designation, however, can only be asserted if the material behaves according to an underpinning of the Weibull behavior, which cannot be assessed using other distribution functions: the size effect on strength.

The size effect is the dependence of the strength on the size of the specimen, in that larger specimens have a higher probability of containing large strength-limiting defects, yielding lower strength values than small specimens tested in the same loading conditions. It is thus not surprising that manufacturers tend to show a liking for advertising strength values obtained from biaxial flexure or 3-point bending (low surface and volume) instead of 4-point bending (large surface and volume). A direct comparison between strength values obtained from sets of specimens having different sizes (or same sizes but different testing jig dimensions, for that matter) is fundamentally inappropriate. A procedure to correct for this is implicit in the Weibull fracture theory, namely, the scaling of the strengths obtained from two different specimen sizes (σ_a and σ_b, for example) can be done by considering their effective volumes ($V_{\text{eff,a}}$ and $V_{\text{eff,b}}$) or surfaces ($S_{\text{eff,a}}$ and $S_{\text{eff,b}}$) according to:

$$\sigma_a = \sigma_b\left(\frac{V_{\text{eff,b}}}{V_{\text{eff,a}}}\right)^{1/m}\qquad(3.3)$$

and

$$\sigma_a = \sigma_b\left(\frac{S_{\text{eff,b}}}{S_{\text{eff,a}}}\right)^{1/m}\qquad(3.4)$$

being m the Weibull modulus. Only then can strength values obtained from different test configurations (e.g., 3- or 4-point bending) and specimens sizes using the same test set-up, be compared. The calculation of the V_{eff} and S_{eff} of standardized uniaxial bending configurations is given in Ref. [14]. For other, more complex configurations, this has to be done numerically. An illustration of the size effect on strength is shown in Fig. 3.2 for two materials, where test specimens prepared in the same way (regarding cutting and polishing) were tested in biaxial flexure (both in disc and in plate geometries) having a small effective surface, and in 4-point bending with a larger effective surface [15]. Using Eq. (3.4), strength vs. effective surfaces plots are constructed, with the center lines being the estimations based on the Weibull moduli ($-1/m$), and the uncertainty lines being the 90% confidence intervals. In an ideal agreement with the Weibull theory, the center blue, red, and black prediction lines should align, though falling within the uncertainty range suffices.

For the material IPS e.max® CAD, the Weibull behavior conforms sufficiently well for the range of tested specimen sizes. Though, it deviates strongly from an expected Weibull behavior for the material Vitablocs Mark® II, with the small specimens showing lower strength than predicted by the behavior of the large specimen (or vice versa). This can be a true effect due to completely different flaw populations occurring at different size scales, or an artifact of the testing methodology. In this case, it was probably due to the latter, once the small specimens were cut out of small blocks (I14), whereas the large specimens were cut out of large blocks (I40); they cannot really be compared (unless small specimens from I40 blocks would confirm this), but this exposes how, despite being compositionally the same material, the fabrication process of different block sizes can create different flaw size distributions. For the material IPS e.max® CAD, also two different block sizes were used, but here the fabrication process does not consist of sintering uniaxially compacted milled glass powder mixed with milled feldspar crystals mixed to organic binders, but casted glass that is later crystallized—glasses are much more homogeneous.

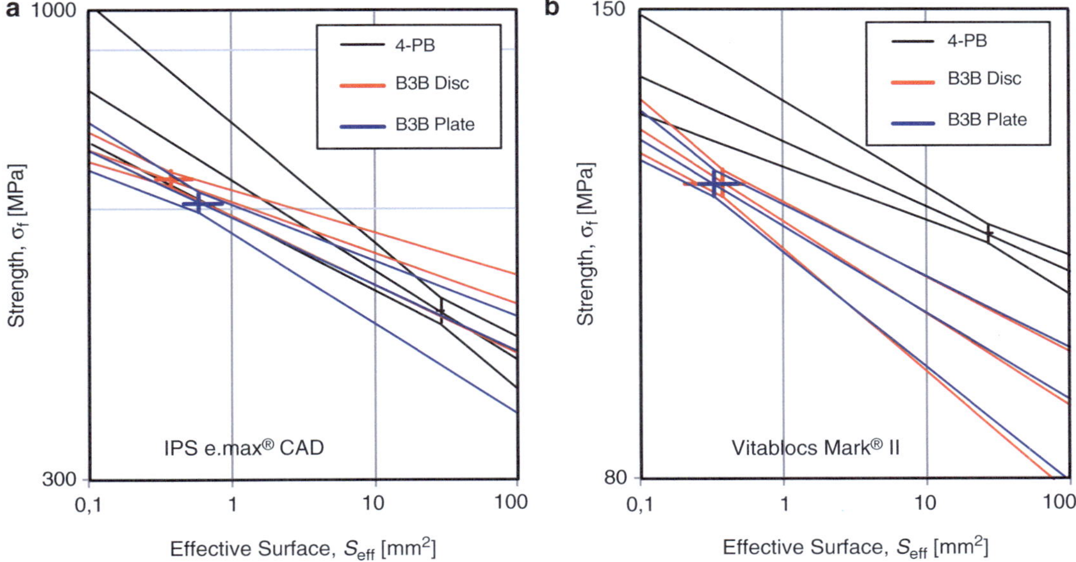

Fig. 3.2 Relationship between the measured strength and the tested effective surface, exposing the compliance to the Weibull behavior in (**a**), but not in (**b**). Results from Ref. [15]

3.1.2 Testing

The above sections preamble the general impression that strength testing constitutes a sensitive procedure entailing a range of practical difficulties that can add up to large errors in individual measured values, consequently affecting the resulting distribution. Apart from the aspects related to specimen fabrication, which were already covered, the strength of ceramic materials will be highly influenced by the test configuration and the peculiarities involved in each test. Although tensile and compressive tests are well established, they are less common, and preference is given for flexural (or "bending") tests either in uniaxial or in biaxial stress state. Uniaxial flexural tests are in 3- or 4-point and are standardized in several norms, such as ASTM C 1161, ISO 17565, ENV 843–1, and ISO 6872, usually for specimens with a cross-section of 4 mm in width and 3 mm in height. The first three standards allow for supporting rollers 20 mm or 40 mm apart (L) and loading rollers in the 4-point configuration having $L/3$ or $L/2$. The dental standard ISO 6872 makes concessions to the usual span lengths defined in the standards it is derived from, allowing for 12 mm for 3-point and 16/8 mm for 4-point bending, meant to facilitate specimen production from materials delivered solely as small CAD/CAM blocks. Though, the miniaturization of test dimensions has shown to intensify geometrical factors that are known to be causes of error, such as fixture articulation, specimen parallelism, friction and wedging, lateral alignment between upper and lower rollers, as well as their plane parallelism [16, 17]. The smaller the testing dimensions, the more refined the testing jig and the more diligent should the operator be [18, 19]. In small bending bars, the chamfering of edges may not be able to remove the large machining damage it once could in wider specimens [20]. Many of the common sources of error can be minimized by: (1) designing jigs that are not fixed to the traverse of the testing machine; (2) using rollers that can shift laterally during the bending of the specimens; (3) allowing for articulation of the upper rollers to adapt better to specimens surfaces that are not

entirely plan-parallel in the length-axis; (4) allowing rollers to tilt, so to compensate for any lack of specimen parallelism in the width-plane; (5) including guides to assure an appropriate alignment between upper and lower parts; etc. One such custom jig has been introduced in Ref. [21], and is shown in Fig. 3.3.

Alternatively, biaxial test configurations offer many advantages that eliminate common drawbacks of uniaxial tests using beams, apart from requiring less material and allowing smaller specimen sizes. The direction of grinding relative to axes of the tensile side of the specimen, of importance when using uniaxial tests, becomes irrelevant, once the stress state becomes equibiaxial, with all defects oriented perpendicular to the tensile direction. Of particular benefit is the non-incorporation of specimen edges under the loaded area, once they hang outside of the sup-

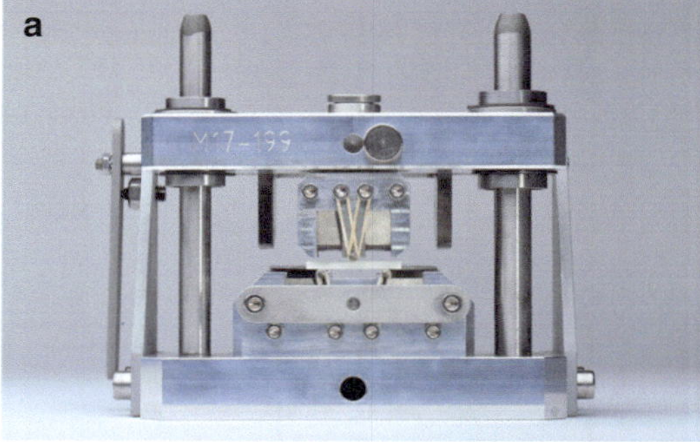

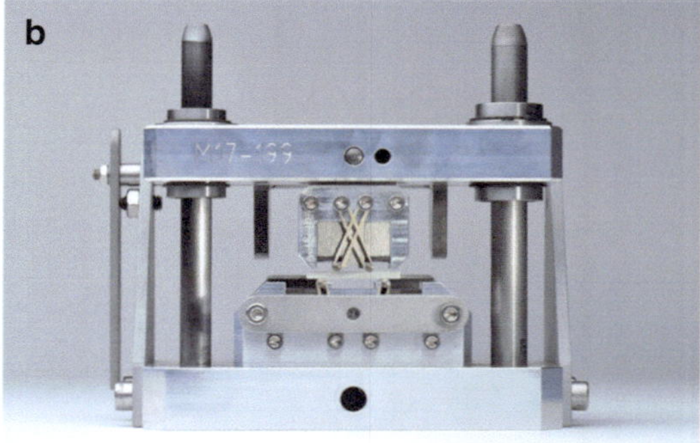

Fig. 3.3 Fully articulated removable jig for 3-point (**a**) and 4-point (**b**) uniaxial bending having ball-bearing lateral guides that assure the alignment of the upper and lower parts of the fixture. In the image, the supporting span measures 20 mm but can be expanded to 40 mm. The loading span of the 4-point fixture has 10 mm in the image, with possibility for setting it to 20 mm

ports. However, some configurations, such as the pin-on-disc test (standardized in ISO 6872), ball-on-ring, ring-on-ring, three-balls-on-three-balls are more sensitive to the plan-parallelism of the specimens once both supporting and loading sides form planes; slightly warped specimens must then be grinded, losing its original surface structure. Biaxial fixtures are also more sensitive to friction at the contact areas/points with the specimen, and the use of an intermediate layer can contribute to error in some tests [22]. An interesting solution to some of these problems of those well-established biaxial tests is the ball-on-three-balls test [23], which allow the loading balls to roll outward during bending of the specimen [24], reducing thereby sliding friction. Due to non-fixed contact points, testing of specimens with flatness deviations up to 16% can be tested without significant loss of accuracy [24]. The test has been expanded for rectangular plates [25, 26], and adapted for sizes relevant for CAD-CAM materials in Ref. [15]. Figure 3.4 illustrates the pin-on-disc set-up within the recommendations of ISO 6872, and the ball-on-three-balls for comparison.

3.2   The Fracture Toughness Concept

As laid out in Sect. 3.1, the dependence of strength on the effective surface/volume of the tested component (specimen size), as well on the preparation procedures dictating the surface quality, make of

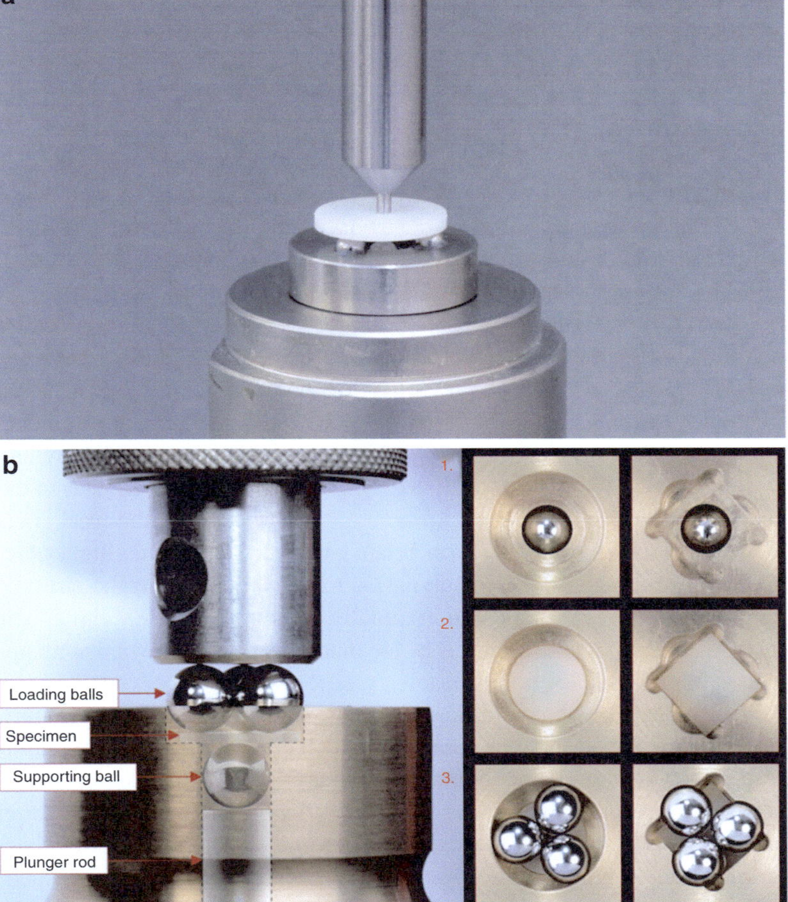

Fig. 3.4 Biaxial flexural test set-ups. (**a**) pin-on-disc and (**b**) ball-on-three-balls for disc and plate geometries. Image (**b**) is reprinted with permission from Elsevier, from Ref. [15]

strength for an unreliable mechanical parameter to be considered as "inherent" material property. Additionally to strength values showing a certain statistical distribution, the model of stress at fracture can communicate us with valuable information on a set of specimens fabricated and processed according to a specific procedure, but fail to replicate for the exact same composition once, for example, finishing steps and testing procedures are changed, if only slightly. Comparisons among laboratories and studies, let alone among testing data supplied by manufacturers, will lead to inevitable confusion if strength alone is to be used as a measure of a material's resistance to fracture. A theoretical model able to fully describe the fracture behavior in terms of an invariant physical quantity, could therefore not rely solely on the stress at fracture. A failure criterion must therefore exist involving some physical quantity in order to fit the meaning of material fracture within a mechanistic framework.

3.2.1 Principles

The most important precept of fracture mechanics, the one which shaped the framework upon which the field developed, is built upon the relationship between the stress applied to a body (σ_{appl}) and the size and shape of the defect (or crack, a) most unfavorably oriented in that stress field, by means of the stress intensity factor K_I (the index I denotes here pure tension mode):

$$K_{I,appl} = \sigma_{appl} Y \sqrt{\pi a_i}, \qquad (3.5)$$

where Y is a correction term related to the geometry of the crack. The crack is said to have an initial length a_i, which could eventually come to grow as $K_{I,appl}$ increases, such as for materials that exhibit some R-curve behavior (see Sect. 3.3), or under fatigue conditions (see Sect. 3.4). The value of $K_{I,appl}$ cannot increase indefinitely: it reaches a maximum at the moment of fracture— it is said to reach *criticality*, or become *critical* (denoted by the subscript c), and $K_{I,appl}$ becomes then K_{Ic}, also known as the *fracture toughness* (FT):

$$K_{Ic} = \sigma_c Y \sqrt{\pi a_c}. \qquad (3.6)$$

That implies that a body fractures catastrophically whether (1) the applied stress reaches a critical value σ_c for a static initial crack size a_i (here there is no crack grown until $\sigma_{appl} = \sigma_c$), or (2) the crack reaches a critical size a_c at some constant or varying applied stress (here there is a so-called *subcritical crack growth* at $\sigma_{appl} < \sigma_c$, with the crack becoming unstoppable at $\sigma_{appl} \geq \sigma_c$). The failure criterion is $K_{I,appl} \geq K_{Ic}$. Between a_i and a_c, if there is any crack growth before K_{Ic} is reached, the crack is said to grow *subcritically*, or *stably*, a behavior that will be addressed in the next sections.

Equation (3.6) is known as the Griffith–Irwin relation, developed by Irwin in 1957 [27] and built upon the works of Inglis [28] and Griffith [29] in the early twentieth century, despite early contributions to the field being reported back to 1907 by Wieghardt [30]. Inglis worked independently on the idea that flaws are responsible for stress concentrations in loaded bodies, and detailed the stress field at the tip of an elliptical opening, which increases at the tip with its half-length and sharpness, i.e., $\propto \sqrt{a/r}$, where r is the flaw tip radius. Griffith developed later an energy approach based on the equilibrium between the stored elastic energy in the loaded body and the surface energy needed for creating two new surfaces during crack growth, establishing a proportionality between fracture stress and the inverse square root of crack length, i.e., $\sigma_c \propto a_c^{-1/2}$. The stored energy release rate G, introduced by Griffith, equates to the two new surface areas created by the crack, i.e., $G = 2\gamma$ (although orders of magnitude higher are expected in practice), and relates to the stress intensity factor of Irwin by $G = K^2/E$, with E being the Young's modulus. A useful review with applicability to dental bonded interfaces can be found in Ref. [31].

The K-concept turned out to be extremely convenient, holding not only a theoretical but also a practical significance, as it serves as the basis of laboratorial tests for obtaining the fracture toughness or any other dynamic behaviors of the stress intensity factor, such as R-curve measurements and crack growth velocity relationships. In many standardized fracture toughness tests, σ_c in Eq. (3.6) is substituted by the solution for the fracture stress under the loading condition in question, be that 3- or 4-point uniaxial bending, biaxial flexure, tension, etc. The rearrangement of Eq. (3.6) can be very useful in practice, enabling one to derive the stress at failure for a specific component if K_{Ic} and a_c are known:

$$\sigma_c = \frac{K_{Ic}}{Y\sqrt{\pi a_c}}, \qquad (3.7)$$

or to calculate the critical defect size if K_{Ic} and σ_c are available:

$$a_c = \frac{1}{\pi} \times \left(\frac{K_{Ic}}{Y\sigma_c} \right)^2. \qquad (3.8)$$

To account for stress concentrators, defects, and cracks assuming different shapes, a geometry factor is needed to correct for that effect, including the influence of loading conditions. This is accomplished by the Y term in Eqs. (3.5–3.8), which can be estimated to $Y = 1.1215$ for a straight-through edge crack, such as a surface scratch from grinding procedure, $Y = 2/\pi$ for a penny-shaped defect embedded in the bulk, and $Y = 2\sqrt{2/\pi}$ for penny-shaped crack touching the surface [32]. Should the π term be already included in the estimation of Y, it must not be accounted for twice. Specific crack geometries for individual testing conditions are usually made available in testing standards.

3.2.2   Testing

Testing of FT is undoubtedly a very sensitive undertaking, and detailed aspects of tests and procedures have been extensively addressed in Refs. [21, 33–41].

The majority of FT tests are nothing more than quasi-static strength tests, with the corresponding specimens having an additional artificially fabricated pre-crack or notch. Summed to all the complexities related to testing of strength mentioned in Sect. 3.1.2, FT testing introduces practical difficulties involving the production of a defect by the operator, of sufficient sharpness for it to behave as a realistic crack, and having a predefined geometry that can be evaluated analytically.

Although natural defects could be used, artificial cracks are preferred to control size and shape, but also to provide for test standardization. The geometry factor Y must therefore be calculated separately, since different cracks, specimen geometries, and loading conditions change depending on the test method. Generally, standardized crack geometries for FT testing are whether (1) *through-the-thickness cracks* or (2) *surface cracks*. The crack geometry in (1) is planar extending from one side of the specimen to the other, for methods such as the single-edge-V-notched-beam (SEVNB), single-edge-pre-cracked-beam (SEPB), compact tension (CT), double cantilever beam (DCB), double torsion (DT); or start from inner holes such as in the double-cleavage-drilled-compression (DCDC). The crack geometry in (2) is usually restricted to the tensile surface of the specimen, usually being created by indentation, such as in the surface-crack-in-flexure (SCF) or in the Vickers-indentation-strength (VIS) methods, both of which are subjected to strength testing. A special case is the Vickers-indentation-fracture (VIF) method, which forgoes the fracture of the specimen and seizes solely on the length of the crack emanating from the corners of a Vickers impression [42].

A special crack type is created in the chevron-notched-beam (CNB) test and variations thereof, consisting of a double-notch creating a V-shaped cross-section that concentrates the tensile stress at its tip during loading, from where a natural crack nucleates and grows subcritically for a certain length up to the point where the specimen fractures [43]. This pop-in crack is a validity requirement for the test, ascertained from the load displacement diagram, which should show a change in specimen compliance moments before fracture. An equipment sensitive enough to small changes in strain directly in the specimen (such as strain-gages, mechanical or optical extensometers) is usually necessary, increasing the complexity of the test. For some materials, the pop-in crack is difficult to obtain, requiring the lowering of the loading rate, or the pre-damaging of the notch tip by successive compressive loading. In Fig. 3.5, the cross-section of a fractured CNB specimen is illustrated, with the damaged tip shown in higher magnification.

The simplicity of specimen production and testing usually dictates the popularity of methods, with factors such as cost, effort, and need for special equipment determining method selection. Unfortunately, most of the popular methods carry the highest degree of uncertainty and sources of error. In ascending order of simplicity, one could attempt a classification of the aforementioned methods as following: VIF > VIS > SEVNB > CT > SCF > CNB > SEPB > DT > DCB > DCDC. This ranking is also that of popularity. In terms of precision and accuracy, that ranking looks rather like: IF < IS < SEVNB ≡ CT < DT < SCF ≡ CNB ≡ SEPB ≡ DCB ≡ DCDC. An excellent compromise between laboriousness and reliability can be reached by using the methods SCF, CNB, and SEPB, incidentally the ones standardized in ASTM C 1421 [44], or in ISO 18756 [45], ISO 24370 [46], and ISO 15732 [47], respectively.

The VIF method [42, 48–50] requires little material and little effort, serving well for quick comparison between experimental batches, but it is deemed to deliver values that do not tend to match those obtained by more reliable methods [51, 52]. Despite evidenced shortcomings [53],

VIF continues to be widely used. The VIS method requires that a Vickers indentation be placed on a defined specimen geometry for strength testing, and no crack measurement is needed; the obtained values do not always match that of other more established methods [54]. The reason might lie in the fact that the residual stress surrounding the plastically deformed impression site, as well as other cracks, are not removed, which can influence the stress state of the median crack. A procedure to remove this damage zone is prescribed in the SCF method by polishing off some specific depth of a Knoop indentation so to maintain only a subsurface semielliptical median crack for which a Y value can be directly calculated [55]. Recently, improved derivations of the Y factor for such crack geometries have been made available [56, 57]. The SCF can be used in the standardized form of beams under four-point bending or under biaxial flexure [58]. Figure 3.6 shows the morphology of a Knoop impression resulting in oblique lateral cracks developing into the subsurface and the median crack orthogonal to the surface, before and after the polishing procedure.

The taken-to-be pre-cracks in SEVNB and CT specimens are usually produced by a double-notch technique, in which a saw cut is produced followed by a razor blade used with polishing pastes to produce an extension having a sharper tip in front of the notch. However, for the notch root not to interfere in the stress state at the tip, the length of this extension should be larger than

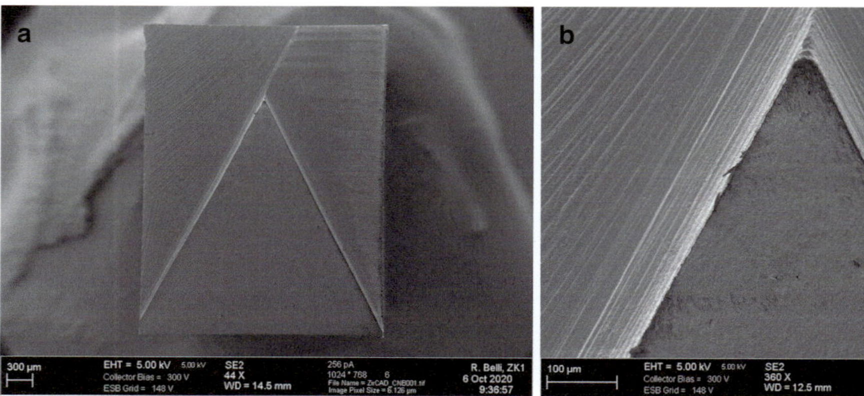
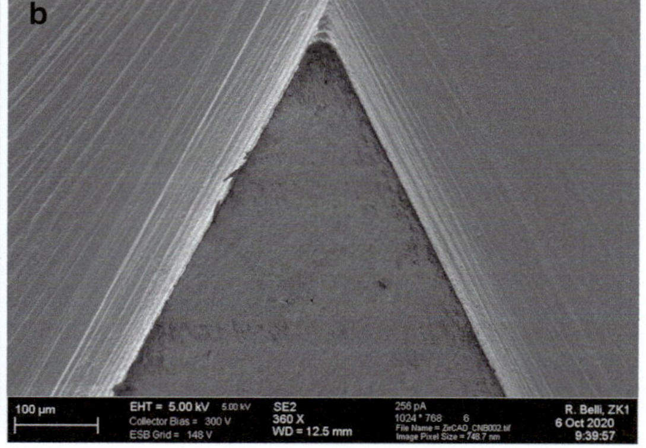

Fig. 3.5 Scanning electron microscopy of (**a**) the V-shape cross-section of a fractured CNB specimen, and (**b**) the damaged tip by successive compression

1.5 times the radius of the sawed notch root [60]. The problem lies in obtaining a sharp tip in this razor blade extension, as its radius should have a comparable size or be smaller than the size of the typical microstructural feature. That radius should not be larger than 1.5–3 times the average grain/crystal size [61]. For materials having sub-

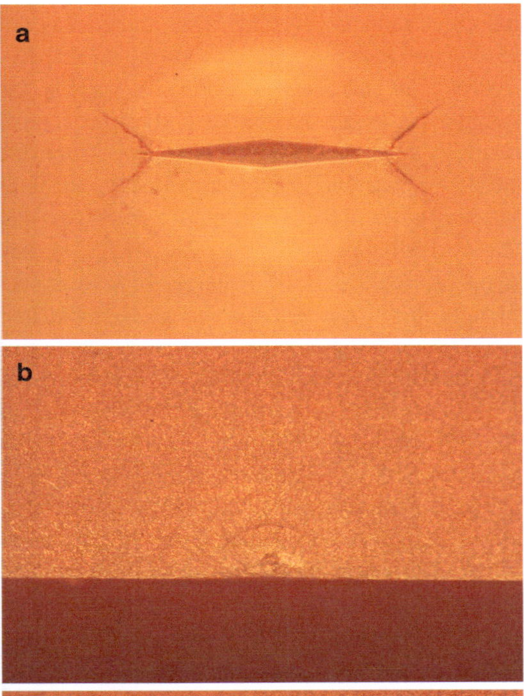

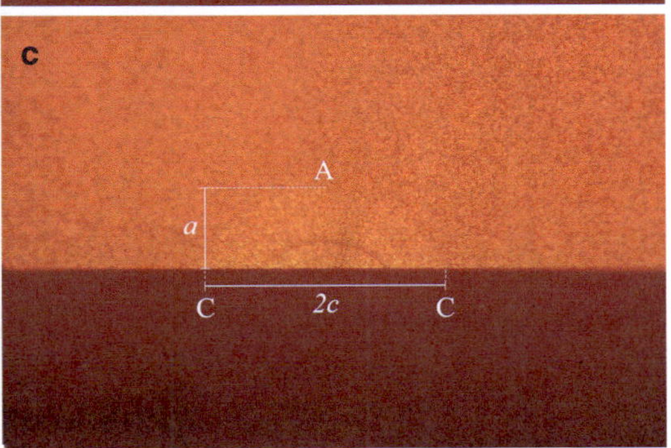

Fig. 3.6 Production of a surface pre-crack for the SCF method. (**a**) Knoop impression showing lateral cracks (lighter halo above and below the impression); (**b**) morphology of the subsurface damage zone plus median crack of an unpolished Knoop-crack system and; (**c**) a fracture surface of a polished Knoop indentation with a remaining median semielliptical crack of length $2c$ and depth a. Taken from Reprinted with permission from Elsevier [59]

micrometric second phases, a mechanically produced sharpened notch will almost invariably be too blunt in order for it to behave like a real crack, leading to the overestimation of the measured fracture toughness. For mostly amorphous materials, such as glasses and low crystallinity glass-ceramics, only atomically sharp (natural) pre-cracks are appropriate. Alternatives to solve this problem are (1) to induce a natural fatigue pre-crack at the tip of the notch—an impractical procedure difficult to reproduce—and (2) to use expensive techniques such as femtosecond laser ablation [62–65].

Apart from sources of error related to inappropriate testing fixtures and loading configuration, accuracy in FT testing suffer mostly due to failure in producing geometrically acceptable pre-cracks (here standard requirements should be respected), such as blunted notch tips (e.g., SEVNB and CT), oblique cracks (e.g., SEVNB and SEPB), insufficiently removed indentation damage (e.g., IS and SCF), stress states not in pure mode-I tension (e.g., DT), occurrence of subcritical crack growth during the test (e.g., CNB), among others. The variability of obtained values within a set of specimens is stochastically distributed (most probably related to variations in microstructure and density along the crack path), showing no theoretical basis for being treated using Weibull statistics [66].

3.3 R-Curve Behavior

The maximum value of $K_{\mathrm{I,appl}}$, i.e., K_{Ic}, should—theoretically—be a constant. For most brittle amorphous materials, such as silicate glasses, it is, and K_{Ic} remains to be considered a material-specific property. Meaning, in a quasi-static test in an inert controlled environment, a pre-crack of size a_{i} does not extend before K_{Ic} is reached upon loading, so that $a_{\mathrm{i}} = a_{\mathrm{c}}$. Though for brittle materials presenting second phases, and ductile materials exhibiting considerable plastic deformation upon fracture, the formerly critical value K_{Ic} has been shown to increase for growing cracks: $K_{\mathrm{I,appl}} = f(\Delta a)$. $K_{\mathrm{I,appl}}$ is a function of the change in crack length. That is, a pre-crack grows stably in a subcritical K_I-regimen before the crack becomes unstoppable (critical). In a typical plot of applied $K_\mathrm{I,appl}$ against change in a (Δa), what we see is a steep curve that tends to become flatter with the growing crack, the so-called *crack growth resistance curve*, or *R-curve*. In simple terms, the material imposes some resistance as the crack propagates, until a certain plateau $K_\mathrm{I,max}$ is reached. Technically, the crack requires extra energy from the system to continue to grow, in the form of extra applied load.

In materials having heterogeneous microstructural arrangements along the crack path, the R-curve can seem to assume an exponential shape, such as when a crack propagates from the surface to the inner enamel layer [67]. This is an artefact due to the anisotropic gradient present through the thickness of the specimen. In some isotropic homogeneous materials, the R-curve can also appear linear. Such materials are referred to as "*R-curve materials*"; they are no "*smart materials*" in the sense of the word, since the material is not learning anything. There is simply some sort of energy dissipation as the crack interacts with the microstructure ahead or behind it [68–73].

The virtue of R-curve therefore implies that some shielding of the crack tip stress intensity factor $K_\mathrm{I,tip}$ occurs during the extension of a crack, by an amount $K_\mathrm{I,sh}$ at each new crack increment, i.e., $K_\mathrm{I,sh}(\Delta a)$. The subscript "sh" is generalized, and can be exchanged to refer to the known mechanism in operation, such as "br" for crack bridging. The applied K_I by an external load, $K_\mathrm{I,appl}$, becomes:

$$K_\mathrm{I,appl} = K_\mathrm{I,tip} - K_\mathrm{I,sh}\left(\Delta a\right) \qquad (3.9)$$

with $K_\mathrm{I,sh}$ being negative—and increases up to some critical crack length a_c, when the unstable critical condition sets in [11]:

$$K_\mathrm{I,appl} = K_\mathrm{I,max}, \quad \frac{\partial K_\mathrm{I,appl}}{\partial a} = \frac{\partial K_\mathrm{IR}}{\partial a}, \qquad (3.10)$$

also called the tangent condition. Unfortunately, R-curves are difficult to measure accurately, especially if $K_\mathrm{I,max}$ is reached already after very short crack growth (typical for short semi-elliptical

cracks and small specimen sizes; typical lab universal testing machines are too compliant to detect and unload the specimen fast enough so to arrest the crack before instability. Due to such testing problems, allusions to possible R-curve effects can be inferred from indirect evidences. From Eq. (3.10) it holds that the obtained K_Ic-value, as measured in a quasi-static test, should be higher for specimens of the same material having longer initial crack lengths [74, 75]. If the material is not really an R-curve material (also called K_Ic-*material*, or *flat R-curve material*), varying the initial crack length using a set of specimens, must result in a single K_Ic-value. Therefore, from one single fracture toughness test geometry, one cannot really tell if the K_Ic-value obtained from the standard solution represents a K_Ic, a $K_\mathrm{I,max}$, or any $K_\mathrm{I,appl}$ located along the R-curve. It is to expect though, that if the material has an R-curve, and only one test is available, that those geometries allowing high crack extension are due to render K_Ic-values farther along the R-curve [76], such as the Single-Edge-Precracked-Beam and the Chevron-Notched-Beam specimens, as opposed to cracks in the Surface-Crack-in-Flexure method. However, since one cannot know a priori the range of Δa possible for a certain material and specimen geometry, cracks that saturate very quick can result in similar K_Ic-values for different methods, and lead one to conclude that the material has a flat R-curve. To resolve that problem, the crack initiation toughness, K_I0 (the value of $K_\mathrm{I,appl}$ when $a = a_\mathrm{i}$) can be measured using crack opening displacement methods [77–81].

If an accurate measurement of the R-curve is attained, usually by optical methods (direct or indirect) or the compliance method, its shape, its steepness, its range over (Δa), the presence or not of a plateau $K_\mathrm{I,max}$, and the value of $K_\mathrm{I,0}$, are taken as descriptors of the fracture behavior and used for tailoring the microstructure.

It is, however, important to bear in mind, that the same material being tested in different conditions will not exhibit the same shape of the R-curve, such as when type of loading and specimen geometry [76, 82–86]. Also, it is expected that specimens having long initial pre-crack sizes will result in R-curves starting at different points along an R-curve obtained in specimens with short pre-cracks. Therefore, R-curves cannot be taken as reproducible or even as a material parameter.

3.3.1 Shielding Mechanisms

In coarse-grained ceramics [87–89], just as in fiber-reinforced composites [90, 91], the negative (compressive) shielding term $K_{\mathrm{I,sh}}$ is induced by bridging mechanisms in the form of unbroken microstructural ligaments that carry some of the load, alleviating some stress from the crack tip. Only elastic stress components will contribute to $K_{\mathrm{I,br}}$ when the bridging element is a rigid local continuum, which becomes proportional to the Young's modulus of the bridge material. When the toughness of the interface (or grain boundary) is lower than that of the bridging element (such as a particulate, or fiber), debonding can take place instead of the fracture of the bridge. The bridging element can then slide inside its encasing as the crack faces open, making the total bridging stress composed of an elastic and a frictional term: $\sigma_{\mathrm{br,tot}} = \sigma_{\mathrm{br,el}} + \sigma_{\mathrm{br,fr}}$. Consequently, the frictional coefficient between both surfaces and the length of the sliding path increase $\sigma_{\mathrm{br,fr}}$. If there is any

thermal mismatch in strains between particulate and matrix, the friction is enhanced. Consequently, elongated particulates of high aspect ratio, stiffness, and toughness, that are moderately bonded to the matrix, consist of ideal bridging elements [92], since they favor the occurrence of $\sigma_{\mathrm{br,el}}$ and $\sigma_{\mathrm{br,fr}}$. In Fig. 3.7 these mechanisms are illustrated separately and combined.

If there is no debonding and the crack has to deflect along a particulate, it stalls as it has to go around it, in a direction that is not energetically favorable. This induces a high tensile field ahead of the particulate, where a new crack nucleates and has to extend backward. This process results in high energy expenditures, and is shown in Fig. 3.8 as modeled by in Ref. [94]. There, two important geometrical aspects are highlighted: the higher the aspect ratio of the particulate and its angle to the crack plane, generally the higher is the energy consumption, which can be translated in terms of σ_{br}. The R-curve benefits of high aspect ratio grain and a not-so-strong grain boundary adhesion have been demonstrated experimentally [87, 95]. For the lithium disilicate IPS e.max® Press, the orientation of the $\mathrm{Li_2Si_2O_5}$ crystallites at 90° with the crack plane led to a significant R-curve developing over the range of 1.69 MPa $\sqrt{\mathrm{m}}$ (natural defect) up to 2.25 MPa $\sqrt{\mathrm{m}}$

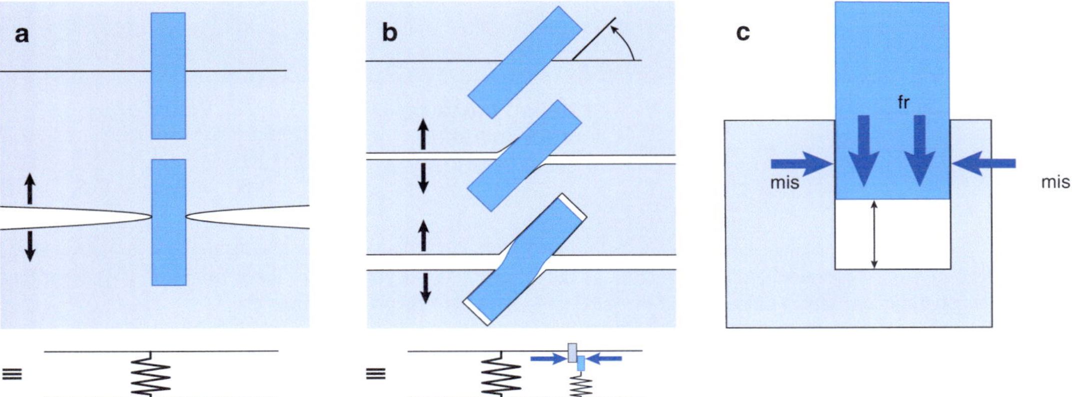

Fig. 3.7 Schematic of the crack bridging mechanism. (**a**) Crack growing passed a bridging element without fracturing or debonding, resulting in a purely elastic component. (**b**) Crack growing passed an angled bridging element with interfacial debonding with subsequent sliding and bending as the crack opening displacement δ increases, creating elastic and frictional components. (**c**) Detail of frictional stress σ_{fr} amplified by mismatch stress σ_{mis} between bridging element and the surrounding matrix. Adapted from Ref. [93]

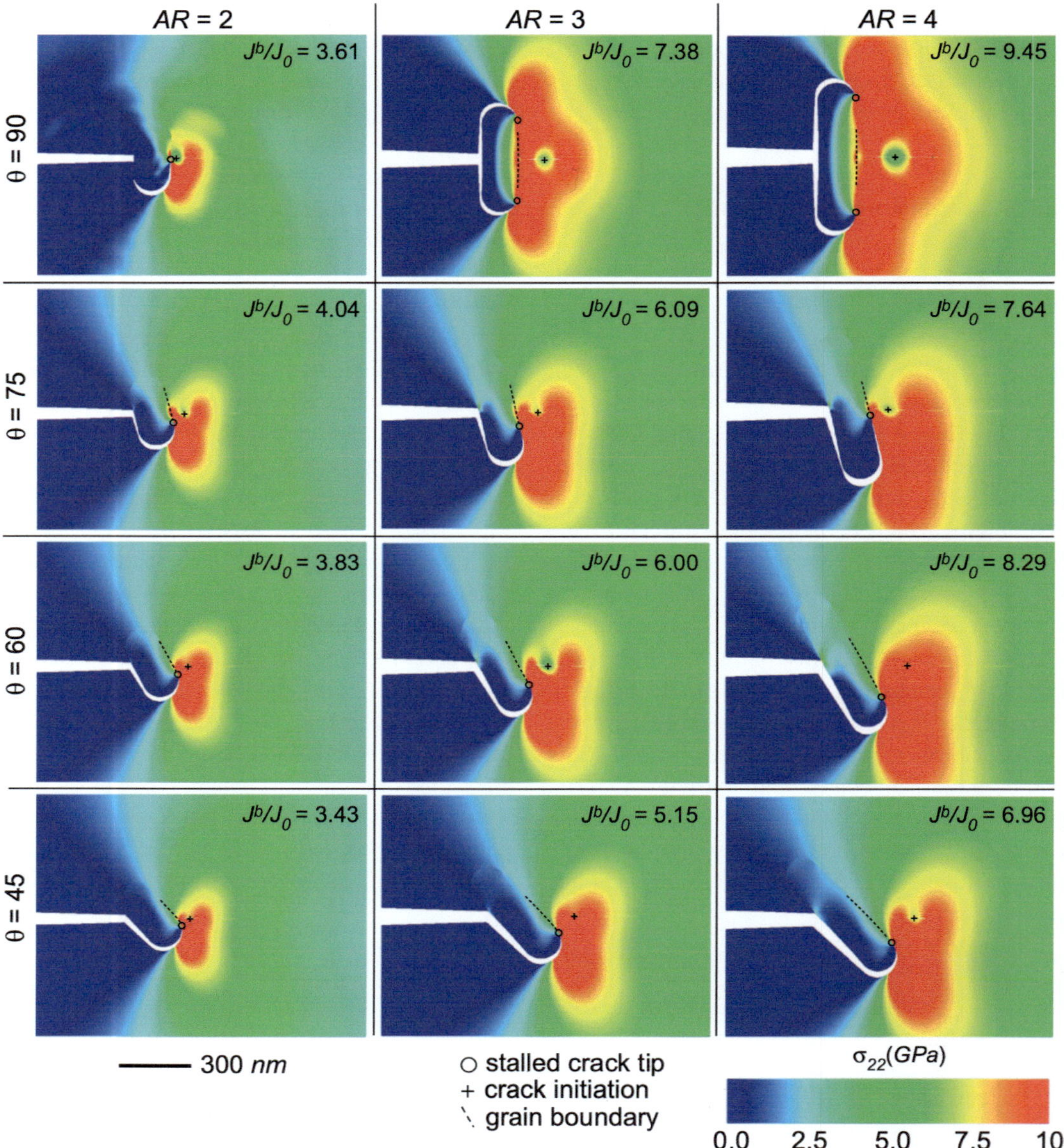

Fig. 3.8 Stress concentrations during crack bridging after deflection around a precipitate as a function of the angle of encounter θ and aspect ratio (AR) of the particulate. J^b/J_0 is the normalized driving force for bridging from the stalled position (circle) to the re-initiation ahead (cross) of the particulate. Taken from Ref. [94]. Reprinted with permission from Elsevier

(CNB specimen) [89]. The high aspect ratio of $Li_2Si_2O_5$ in IPS e.max® Press also resulted in a higher $K_{I,max}$ and a much superior resistance to crack growth in the subcritical regimen than the low aspect ratio crystals in IPS e.max® CAD, even though the latter has a higher degree of crystallinity (61 vol.% vs. 67 vol.%, respectively) [89, 96]. The material Vitablocks Mark II, which contains feldspar crystals of up to 20 μm in size also showed indirect signs of having an R-curve,

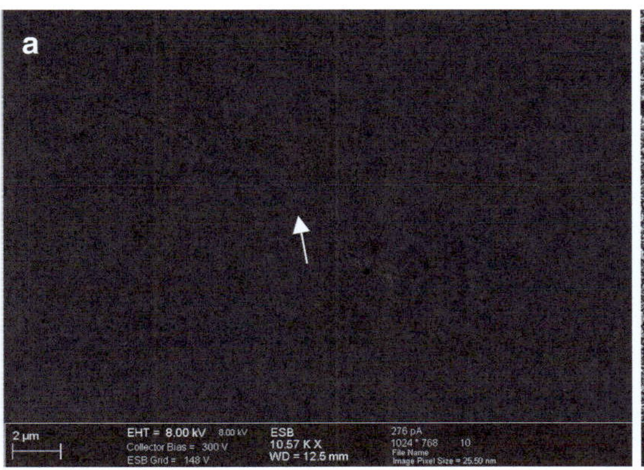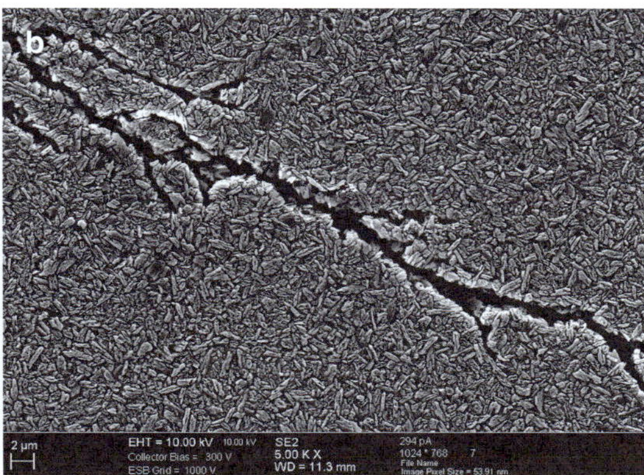

Fig. 3.9 Crack shielding mechanisms seen in developed cracks. (**a**) SEM image in backscattered mode of a crack in IPS e.max® Press showing uncracked ligaments (elastic bridges, black arrows) and interlocking (white arrow). (**b**) SEM image of a crack in etched (5% HF, 10s) IPS e.max® CAD showing multiple crack branching. Taken from Ref. [89]. Reprinted with permission from Elsevier

showing short crack toughness of 0.88 MPa$\sqrt{\text{m}}$ (SCF specimen [59]) and long-crack toughness of 1.19 MPa$\sqrt{\text{m}}$ (SEPB specimen [97]) and 1.23 MPa$\sqrt{\text{m}}$ (CNB specimen [59]).

Other shielding mechanisms acting in dental ceramics, which contribute to the development of R-curve effects are *crack deflection, crack branching, interlocking,* and *transformation toughening*. The latter is characteristic of polycrystalline zirconias containing high amounts of a transformable *t*-phase, especially 2–3Y-TZP, and zirconia-alumina composites, and is dealt with in depth in Sect. 2.3. *Microcracking* in the grains resulting from such phase transformation also seems to produce residual compressive stresses that add to the shielding component [98], but with much lesser effectiveness than the transformation itself [99]. Interlocking occurs often in ceramics with randomly oriented elongated microstructures, and consists of a mechanism that opposes crack opening due to a mechanical obstruction, such as an oblique grain that has been contoured by a crack (see Fig. 3.9a), or debris from broken bridges wedging the crack faces. Crack branching occurs when the microstructure forces the crack to split into different planes (almost parallel), suggestively due to a large microstructural bridge that could not be broken, increasing the crack surface and therefore the energy consumption to create those new

surfaces, which usually leads to the arrest of one of the branches [11] (see Fig. 3.9b).

Crack deflection takes place around tougher precipitates of different sizes, increasing the overall toughness of two-phase materials, but it does not necessarily lead to an R-curve effect unless generating substantial new extra energy consumption during crack growth. That can happen when the microstructure deflects the crack away from the direction of the principal tensile stress—the preferred path of crack growth— forcing it to states of shear loading, which are energetically unfavorable. Examples of such behaviors can be seen in dental enamel and dentin [100–103], and possible in ceramics containing elongated second phases that can be aligned by heat pressing [89, 104, 105].

3.4 Subcritical Crack Growth

Both *flat R-curve* (K_{Ic} exists) or *rising R-curve* behaviors are good descriptors of the fracture process during monotonic loading. But overloading events take place only rarely in real applications (unless the material is too weak from the start), where the service load is usually a fraction of the maximum sustainable load, with unloading intervals happening in a cyclical manner. Even if the applied stress never surpasses the critical stress for K_{Ic} or $K_{I,max}$ to be reached, failure can still occur. In such instances (i.e., where fracture occurs at a clearly lower load), some sort of degradation phenomenon is assumed to have acted implicitly, the so-called "fatigue."

In silicate glasses, and in materials exhibiting a molecular structure formed predominantly of oxide bonds, such as Si-O, Al-O, Li-O, and Zr-O—like most bulk dental ceramics—a specific fatigue mechanism called *stress corrosion-assisted subcritical crack growth* (SCASCG) takes place in the presence of water molecules. At the tip of a crack or defect, where the stress is highly concentrated, the water molecule is loosely attracted to the glass through hydrogen bonding between H^+ and the bridging oxygen in Si-O-Si. Stresses acting opening the crack also induce stretching of local Si-O-Si at the crack tip with accompanying changes in the angles between atomic bonds, which will energetically predispose the donation of a proton from the water molecule to the oxygen in the siloxane bond. Simultaneously, an electron is transferred from the oxygen in the water molecule to the silicon atom. The former Si-O-Si bond is thus disrupted, resulting in two Si-O-H groups at opposing fracture surfaces [106]. Thus, upon stress at the crack tip, oxide bonds are hydrolyzed more easily by water [107]:

$$Si\text{-}O\text{-}Si + H_2O + \text{stress} \rightarrow 2\,Si\text{-}OH + \Delta a, \tag{3.11}$$

resulting in crack extension at stresses lower than the critical stress (subcritical) [108]. Although this process is much more pronounced in silicate glasses, it is also active, though to a lesser extent, in polycrystalline materials such as alumina and zirconia. Oxide bonds such as Al-O-Al and Zr-O-Zr are also disrupted by water molecules under mechanical stress, similarly to the reaction in Eq. (3.11), leading to the degradation of strength over time. When dealing with such materials, the term SCASCG is taken as a synonym of fatigue, in a process also abbreviated as *slow crack growth* (SCG). This process is controlled by how fast new water molecules can reach the crack tip of a growing crack (diffusion process) [109], to which term "slow" in SCG alludes, highlighting the time-dependency of this process. In scenarios of very fast crack propagation (for instance, very near K_{Ic}), such as in impact or high loading rate testing, the water corrosion effect goes to zero, since there is no time for water molecules to reach and react at the crack tip in time.

Here one has to be aware of etymological aspects of the term *subcritical* within a fracture mechanics context. That is, all crack growth taking place before the critical crack size a_c is reached, is termed *subcritical*, or *stable*. At $a \geq a_c$, a crack embedded in a homogeneous global tensile stress field is said to be unstable, that is, it cannot be arrested as it accelerates quickly to very fast velocities and will lead to catastrophic failure. All crack growth during R-curve development is also of the *subcritical* nature; in R-curve materials, the critical condition is $K_{I,appl} \geq K_{IR}$. In dental glassy and oxide ceramics that show no R-curve behavior, any subcritical crack growth is believed to be induced by the SCG phenomenon, in which stable growth of strength-limiting defects takes place at stress intensities below the material's critical stress intensity factor; the critical condition here is $K_{I,appl} \geq K_{Ic}$. In R-curve materials that show SCG, both types of subcritical crack growth take place simultaneously and will contribute to the susceptibility to fatigue (unless SCG is inhibited by controlling the test environment).

The susceptibility to SCG is determined by the mechanical fatigue parameter "n", derived from different loading conditions. The "n" parameter is the exponential term acting on the applied stress intensity factor, driving cracks to grow exponentially, according to the so-called Paris law [109, 110]:

$$v = AK_{I,appl}^n = A^* \left(\frac{K_{I,appl}}{K_{Ic}} \right)^n \tag{3.12}$$

where v is the crack velocity, $K_{I,appl}$ is the applied stress intensity factor A, A^*, and n are fatigue parameters. The parameter n is termed the *crack growth susceptibility parameter*, and is used to characterize how prone a material is to fatigue, and can be obtained from static, dynamic, or cyclic experiments. Low n-values characterize materials with high susceptibility to fatigue and vice versa. In Table 3.1, a sum-mary of experimentally obtained n-values for different dental ceramics is shown according to the test condition employed. One must be aware that, since most fatigue experiments are conducted based on strength testing (uncracked specimens), testing parameters such as loading configuration, specimen size, and surface qual-ity will limit comparison among different studies.

Table 3.1 Summary of selected literature on the SCG parameter n for different dental ceramics obtained using different loading conditions

Dental ceramic	Class	Manufacturer	SCG parameter n	Loading type
IPS e.max® ZirCAD MO	3Y-TZP	Ivoclar-Vivadent	26.7 [111]	Cyclic
YZ cubes		VITA Zahnfabrik	76 [112]	Dynamic
Z-CAD®		Metoxit AG	56.5 [113]	Dynamic
Everest ZS		KaVo	30.15 [114]	Dynamic
Everest ZH (HIP)			28.5 [114]	Dynamic
Zpex		Tosoh	30.8 [115]	Static
			20.9 [115]	Cyclic
Zpex4	4Y-TZP		27.7 [115]	Static
			17.9 [115]	Cyclic
ZpexSmile	5Y-TZP		27.2 [115]	Static
			23.7 [115]	Cyclic
In-Ceram® AL	Polycrystalline alumina	VITA Zahnfabrik	72 [112]	Dynamic
In-Ceram® zirconia	Glass-infiltrated alumina-zirconia		13.1 [116]	Dynamic
In-Ceram® alumina	Glass-infiltrated alumina		31.1 [117]	Dynamic
			36.5 [118]	Static
IPS empress® 2	Lithium disilicate	Ivoclar-Vivadent	17.2 [117]	Dynamic
IPS e.max® press			51.4 [96]	Static
			33.4 [96]	Cyclic
IPS e.max® CAD			19.0 [96]	Static
			9.0 [96]	Cyclic
			15.8 [115]	Static
			10.5 [115]	Cyclic
			8.4 [119]	Dynamic
Suprinity® PC	Lithium (di)silicate	VITA Zahnfabrik	11.2 [119]	Dynamic
			15.5 [111]	Cyclic
Celtra® duo		Dentsply-Sirona	19.5 [111]	Cyclic
IPS e.max® ZirPress	Fluorapatite glass-ceramic	Ivoclar-Vivadent	21.7 [120]	Cyclic
IPS d.Sign®			20.4 [117]	Dynamic
Vitadur® alpha	Aluminosilicate glass	VITA Zahnfabrik	38.4 [116]	Dynamic
VM® 7			36 [112]	Dynamic
VM® 9	Leucite glass-ceramic		44 [112]	Dynamic
IPS empress®		Ivoclar-Vivadent	30.1 [117]	Dynamic
IPS empress® CAD			28.4 [111]	Cyclic
IPS ProCAD®			28 [113]	Dynamic
Vitablocs® mark II	Feldspar-reinforced glass	VITA Zahnfabrik	36.6 [119]	Dynamic
			16.8 [118]	Static
			14.5 [111]	Cyclic
Enamic®	Polymer-infiltrated glass scaffold	VITA Zahnfabrik	29.1 [119]	Dynamic
			27.0 [121]	Static
			28.7 [121]	Cyclic

As seen in Table 3.1, *n*-values of polycrystalline and glass-infiltrated oxide ceramics are comparable to those of glassy systems (apart from isolated studies). Although a trend is difficult to recognize due to methodological differences among experiments, some lithium-based glass-ceramics seem to show the highest susceptibility to SCG (*n*-values <20), with aluminosilicate glasses and leucite-based glass-ceramics usually displaying higher *n*-values (>20). Figure 3.10 offers a comparison of different dental ceramic materials under cyclic loading in water, with the *n*-value being the slope of a *v-K* plot.

In glass-ceramics, since the crack tends to extend mostly through the glass phase, especially in low-crystalline content materials, the chemical composition of the residual glass phase should play an important role in the crack growth rate. Barlet et al. [122], for instance, when studying Na_2O-SiO_2-B_2O_3 systems, found indications implicating the degree of depolymerization of the glass network, rather than the number of Si-O-Si bonds in the crack path, as being responsible for influencing the crack growth rate in the first stage of subcritical crack growth. Other factors such as residual stresses in the residual glass [123] and the pH of the environment [124] have been cited as important aspects influencing the obtained *n*-value. With the increase in crystallinity, interactions between the crack front and the crystal phase become so frequent, that they begin to dominate the resistance to the periodical crack extension, with a ubiquitous R-curve being difficult to deconvolute from the SCG phenomenon (see Sect. 3.4.2). Here, just as in R-curves, the aspect ratio and the orientation of elongated particulates will impose different resistances to the subcritical crack growth, as illustrated in Fig. 3.11. High aspect ratio crystals, especially if oriented orthogonal to the crack growth plane—as a direct effect on the R-curve and little due to SCG—increase the resistance to subcritical crack growth.

Fig. 3.10 Representation of a cyclic loading experiment in specimens with natural defects (polished) in terms of crack velocity vs. the maximum stress intensity factor applied in each specimen, normalized by the material's fracture toughness. The slope of the curve is the cyclic *n*-value, n_c. From Ref. [111]

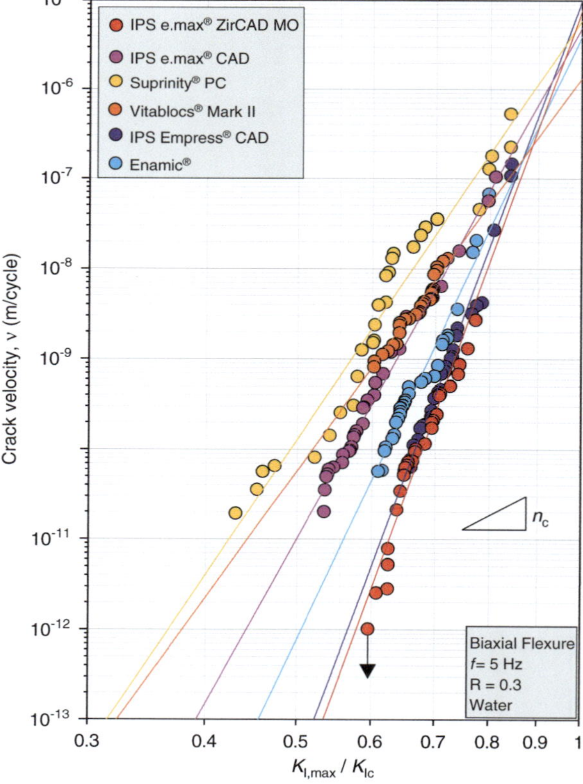

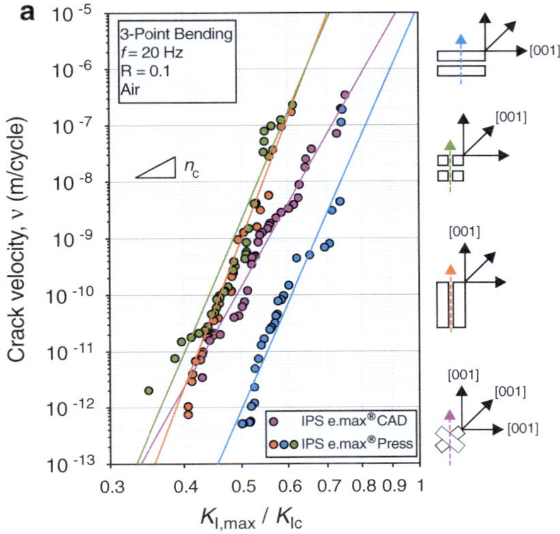
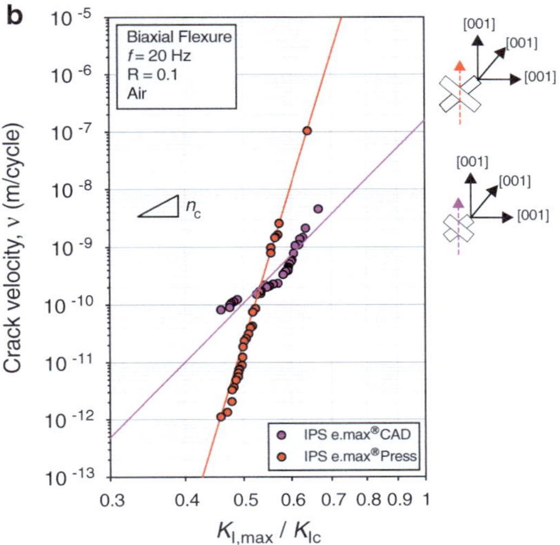

Fig. 3.11 Velocity-K plots of (**a**) uniaxial and (**b**) biaxial cyclic loading experiments in polished lithium disilicate glass-ceramics having comparable crystallinity (vol.% $Li_2Si_2O_5$ crystals) but different crystal aspect ratios. The schematics on the right-hand side of the plots refer to the orientation of the elongated c-axis ([001] direction) in relation to the crack growth plane (colored arrows). In (**a**) different orientations of the $Li_2Si_2O_5$ crystals in IPS e. max® Press show comparable n-values, but the orthogonal orientation shows a shift toward higher stress intensity factors. In (**b**) both materials show random crystal orientation, but the low aspect ratio of crystals in IPS e.max® CAD has a deleterious effect on the n-value. From Ref. [96]

3.4.1 Testing

In order to induce subcritical crack growth to a specimen, two conditions are necessary: time and subcritical stress. If the susceptibility to SCG is to be assessed, a humid testing environment needs to be added to that shortlist. One needs thus to diverge from monotonic tests under fast stress rates in inert environments, the typical conditions used for K_{Ic}-testing. For that, specific testing methodology has been developed within the framework of fracture mechanics, and can be categorized depending on the mode of loading, as static, dynamic, and cyclic tests, which will be addressed below. As will be discussed in Sect. 3.4.2, the combination of two test methods being one a cyclic test will aid in determining the eventual contribution of an R-curve effect or rule it out.

3.4.1.1 Static Tests

In static flexure tests, the specimens are subjected to a pre-defined constant load and the time to fracture is recorded. In tests with one single stress level, a set of specimens taken to be of the Weibull type will show lifetimes according to:

$$P_{F,\text{lifetime static}}\left(t_f\right) = 1 - \exp\left[-\left(\frac{t_f}{t_{f,0}}\right)^{m_s^*}\right], \tag{3.13}$$

with m_s^* (index s for static) being the Weibull modulus obtained from the slope of $\ln(t_f) - \ln(\ln(1/(1 - P_F)))$ plots, with t_0 being the characteristic lifetime. The n-value can be thus derived from the relationship between the Weibull modulus obtained from the static test and from the Weibull modulus m from a set of specimens tested in an inert environment where no SCG can occur:

$$n_\text{s} = \frac{m}{m_\text{s}^*} + 2. \qquad (3.14)$$

For that, the set of inert fast-fracture specimens must contain an equivalent flaw population as the set of specimens tested in the static test, assuring the condition:

$$P_\text{F, inert}\left(\sigma_\text{f}\right) = P_\text{F,static}\left(t_\text{f}\right). \qquad (3.15)$$

Though, a more conventional evaluation of the static fatigue behavior of ceramics subjects several sets of specimens (number of specimens $X \geq 20$) to different stress levels, and requires no inert fast-fracture data. From the fracture mechanics relation of lifetime [110]:

$$t_\text{f} = B\sigma_\text{inert}^{n-2}\sigma^{-n}, \qquad (3.16)$$

the n-value can be obtained from the linear regression of the plot $\log(t_\text{f})$ vs. $\log(\sigma)$ having the slope $= -n$, with the parameter $B\sigma_\text{inert}^{n-2}$ being used to find the crack velocity A^* parameter in Eq. (3.12), through [110]:

$$B = \frac{2K_\text{Ic}^2}{A^*Y^2\left(n-2\right)}. \qquad (3.17)$$

3.4.1.2 Dynamic Tests

In the dynamic flexural test, the time dependency of the fracture stress in materials susceptible to SCG is explored by subjecting comparable sets of specimens to fracture tests at varying stress rates [125]:

$$dt = d\sigma / \dot{\sigma}. \qquad (3.18)$$

The more time is given for the water species to react at the crack tip, the lower is the obtained strength. By plotting $\log(\sigma_\text{f})$ vs. $\log(d\sigma/dt)$ of at least 4 sets of strength measurements, the slope through the median values (or characteristic strength values) gives $1/n + 1$. Each set must contain ≥ 20 specimens. The test benefits from including a very low-stress rate, despite the time expenditure taken. Performing tests in an inert environment at a high-stress rate sets an upper limit to assure that the tests in water at higher stress rates are still showing stress rate depen-

dence; the parameters must be obtained from the linear part of the curve, and not including a higher stress rate in the transition region to the upper limit. Figure 3.12 shows an example of such a plot.

3.4.1.3 Cyclic Tests

As opposed to applications where materials are always subjected to some type of constant load (such as buildings, which are mostly statically loaded in the vertical axis), the oral environment imposes varying periodical loads to restorative materials, making cyclic tests of obvious relevance. Figure 3.13 depicts the parameters that define a period in a typical sinusoidal stress profile $\sigma(t)$ in stress-controlled tests:

$$\sigma\left(t\right) = \sigma_\text{m} + \sigma_\text{a}\sin\left(\frac{2\pi t}{\lambda}\right) \qquad (3.19)$$

with σ_a being the stress amplitude and σ_m the mean stress; the test frequency is $1/\lambda$. The minimum applied stress σ_min and the maximum applied stress σ_max define the R-ratio ($R = \sigma_\text{min}/\sigma_\text{max}$), which can vary from -1 (for $\sigma_\text{min} = \sigma_\text{max}$, with $\sigma_\text{m} = 0$ in pure alternating load), to $-1 \leq R < 1$. Typical relevant

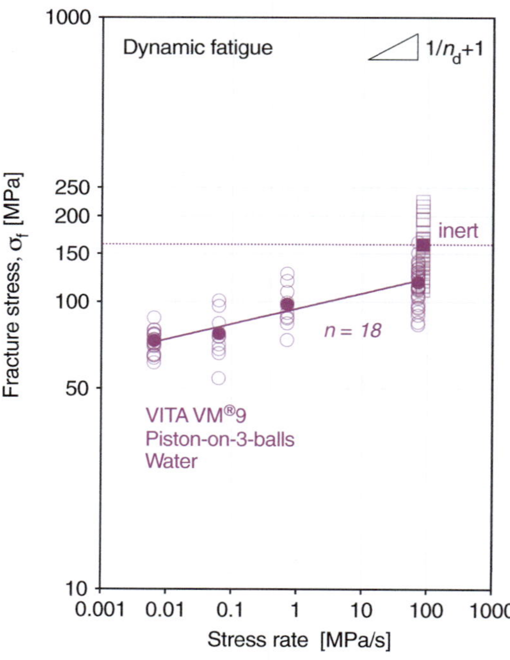

Fig. 3.12 Obtainment of the n-value from dynamic fatigue test in water by means of sets of specimens tested at different stress rates. From Ref. [123]

R-ratios are ≤ 0.5, since $R = 1$ is the case of static loading. The usual representation of cyclical crack growth is made through the change in crack length a, per cycle N, da/dN, plotted against the change in applied stress intensity factor ΔK_{I} or against $K_{I,max}$, normalized of not by the fracture toughness; these are the so-called v-K plots (crack growth rate curves). From such plots, one can also determine the threshold value of K, K_{th}, under which no crack growth occurs, or are too slow to be of practical relevance.

In K-controlled tests, σ is substituted by K in Fig. 3.13, and requires that the crack size is known during crack growth, either by way of (1) performing the test under a microscope (for macroscopic cracks) or (2) tracing the specimen compliance during crack growth (for microscopic cracks). In such tests, like the double-torsion test, the crack velocity v-$K_{I,appl}$ plot is built from one single crack covering slow to high velocities, whether in static or cyclic loading.

If the more complex method of specimen compliance cannot be performed, the representation of the cyclic fatigue behavior for specimens with small natural cracks through da/dN-K_{I} curves can be derived indirectly. This is done by performing cyclic loading experiments in a set of specimens taken as identical to those that are used to determine fast-fracture (inert) strength under the same loading set-up, according to the method described by Fett et al. [126]. The prerequisite is that both sets of specimens have identical flaw populations, in order for the scatter of lifetime to be related to the scatter in the strength data for specimens with corresponding rankings. For that to be fulfilled, one should fabricate spec-

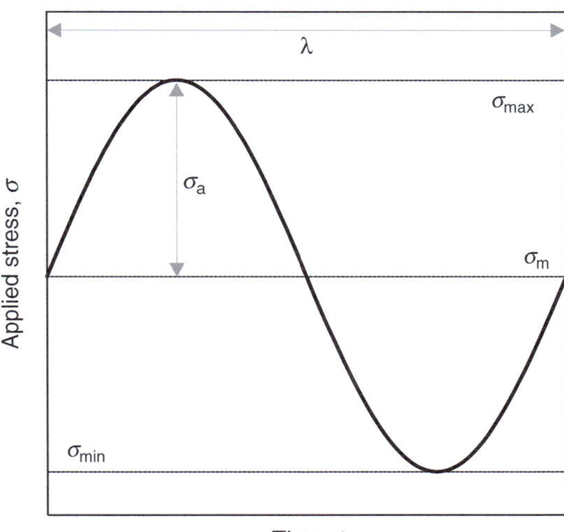

Fig. 3.13 Graphical representation of one period λ in a cyclic loading experiment

imens from both sets (inert and cyclic) together and assign them randomly to one or to the other group. This method assumes that the critical defect leading to fracture at 1 cycle in each fast-fracture specimen is also the one that would grow to criticality (and cause fracture) in a corresponding specimen subjected to lower, but cyclic loading. That is, the crack size in the specimen that fractures under the highest stress in the quasi-static inert test (within a set of specimens) should be equivalent to the crack size in the specimen that survives the longest (in a set having the same number of specimens), and *vice-versa*. Under that assumption, both data scatter, that is, from inert (σ_f) and lifetime (N_f) experiments, follow then a similar failure probability determined by a Weibull distribution, such as:

$$P_{F,\ inert}\left(\sigma_{f}\right) = 1 - \exp\left[-\left(\frac{\sigma_{f}}{\sigma_{0}}\right)^{m}\right], \tag{3.20}$$

and

$$P_{F,\text{lifetime cyclic}}\left(N_{f}\right) = 1 - \exp\left[-\left(\frac{N_{f}}{N_{f,0}}\right)^{m_{c}^{*}}\right]. \tag{3.21}$$

For each material, the Weibull shape parameters m and $m_c{}^*$ (index c for cyclic), and the scale parameters σ_0 and $N_{f,0}$ are determined from $\ln(\sigma_f$ or $N_f)$—$\ln\ln(1/(1 - P_F))$ plots. Both data sets are ranked increasingly and plotted in an auxiliary diagram as $\log(\sigma_{max}/\sigma_{f,i})$ vs. $\log(N_{f,i}\sigma^2{}_{max})$, where the index i stands for the individual values of strength and fatigue specimens. The slope of the resulting linear fitting is used to calculate v, according to [126]:

$$v = -\frac{2K_{Ic}^2}{N_{f,i}\sigma_{f,i}^2 Y^2}\frac{d\log\left(\sigma_{max}/\sigma_{f,i}\right)}{d\log\left(N_{f,i}\sigma_{max}^2\right)}. \quad (3.22)$$

The maximum stress intensity factor $K_{I,max}$ at σ_{max} for the individual inert strength specimens are obtained using the Griffith-Irwin relation:

$$K_{I,max} = \sigma_{max}Y\sqrt{a_{f,i}} = \frac{\sigma_{max}}{\sigma_{f,i}}K_{Ic}, \quad (3.23)$$

where K_{Ic} is the fracture toughness tested in oil at fast loading rates measured preferentially using a surface crack method. For ground specimens, a geometric factor Y of 1.12 can be used, or 1.3 for polished specimens. The resulting v-K curves are straight and correspond to Region I of the Paris Law behavior, such as in Figs. 3.10 and 3.11. In this method, only one fixed stress level for the lifetime experiments is needed, although the combination of two or more stress levels (for extra sets of specimens) can improve the accuracy of the fitting, and should fall within the same trend.

The n-values can be also be obtained by the relationship between the Weibull moduli of inert strength (m) and lifetime, just as with static tests, using [110]:

$$n_c = \frac{m}{m_c^*} + 2, \quad (3.24)$$

with m and $m_c{}^*$ corrected by a bias factor $b(X) \approx \tanh^{1.87}(X - 3.855/0.678)^{0.21375}$ [127], related to the number X of tested samples. Figure 3.14 illustrates the above-described approaches using two different stress levels.

Alternatively to those mechanistic methods, a more phenomenological approach is the Stress-Cycle curve, or S-N curve, which does not require a set of quasi-static strength specimens, but at least two different stress levels. A straight line through the two datasets is obtained in a log $\Delta\sigma$ or $\log(\sigma_{max})$ vs. $\log(N_f)$, with the slope being $-1/n$ (see Fig. 3.15). If the material is known to be Weibull distributed, the fitting can be done through the shape parameter σ_0, otherwise through the median values (also if a reduced number of specimens are used); a slightly different slope is expected.

If only lifetimes stemming from static tests t_{fs} are available, they can be used to predict cyclic lifetimes, using [128]:

$$t_{fc} = g\left(n,\sigma_a/\sigma_m\right)^{-1}\left(\frac{\sigma_s}{\sigma_m}\right)^n t_{fs} \quad (3.25)$$

with σ_s the stress level used in the static test, σ_a the stress amplitude, and σ_m the mean stress used in the cyclic test, being the function $g(n,\sigma_a/\sigma_m)$ determined by:

$$g\left(n,\sigma_a/\sigma_m\right) = \frac{1}{\lambda}\int_0^\lambda\left[\sigma(t)/\sigma_m\right]^n dt. \quad (3.26)$$

If there is no *cyclic fatigue effect* (see Sect. 3.4.2), the predicted t_{fc} should equal the measured t_{fs}, else should t_{fc} predictions be shifted toward higher lifetimes (prediction too high).

Another relevant method for dental restoratives is the contact cyclic fatigue wear test (ball on surface with lateral sliding), which simulates some aspects of the mechanics of mastication by incorporating contact stress fields and friction. Unlike in uniaxial contact fatigue, the incorporation of a tangential component induces shear stresses at the contact surface, with compressive stresses induced at the front of the path and tensile stresses at the trailing edge [129]. Cracks that form into the subsurface have a cone-like geometry, and are called *cone-cracks*; under uniaxial load, two concentric cones are formed: an outer with low angle to the surface and an inner with higher angle. In sliding contact mode, a dense population of partial cone-cracks are generated at

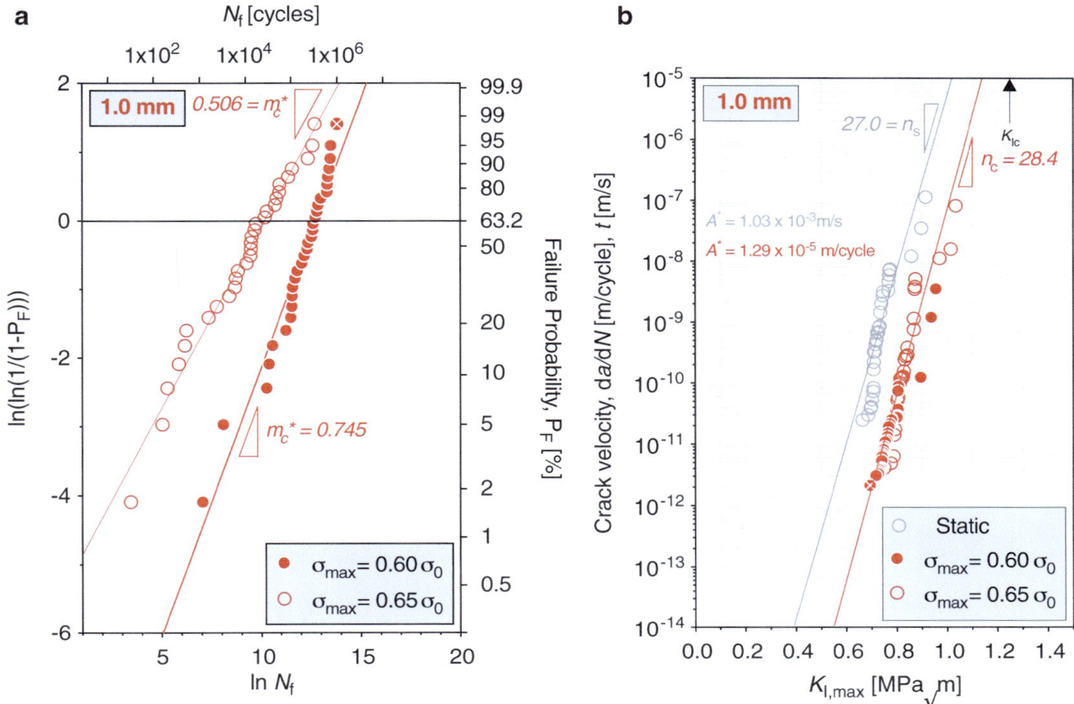

Fig. 3.14 Cyclic crack growth experiments under biaxial flexure ($f = 10$ Hz, $R = 0.3$) for the material Enamic® performed in two different stress levels represented in different forms: (**a**) Weibull distribution and (**b**) v-K plot. Taken from Ref. [121]. Reprinted with permission from Elsevier

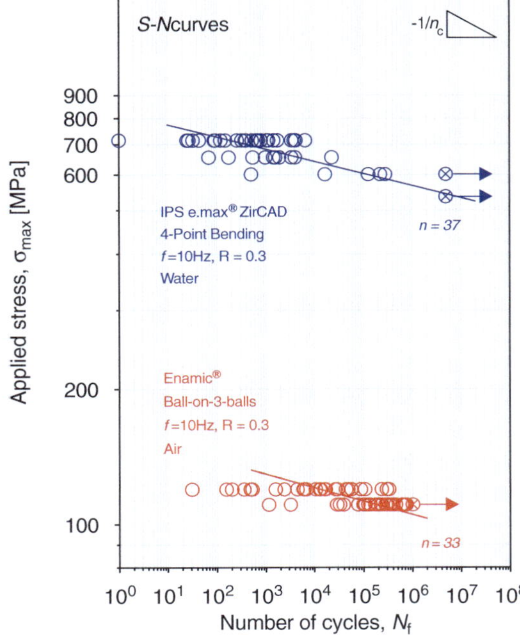

Fig. 3.15 S-N curves of the zirconia IPS e.max® ZirCAD MO and the hybrid composite Enamic®, with the straight line being a fit through the median values at each stress level

the rear of the sliding path [129]. High coefficients of friction lead to steeper angle of these cracks with the surface [130], with frictional stresses increasing as material debris are trapped at the interface. Cone-cracks tend to grow fast at the initial stages of fatigue, aided by hydraulic pumping of water [131], then slowing down at deeper regions when they grow out of the high tensile stress field, which also decreases as the contact area increases (due to a wear scar). Ultimately, the friction coefficient, the elastic modulus, and the fracture toughness [132] control how fast contact cone-cracks evolve. In Fig. 3.16, the surface and subsurface damages to three different restorative materials are shown.

3.4.2 The Effect of R-Curve

In predominantly amorphous glasses (such as some dental veneering ceramics), stress corrosion acts alone. In ceramics toughened by second

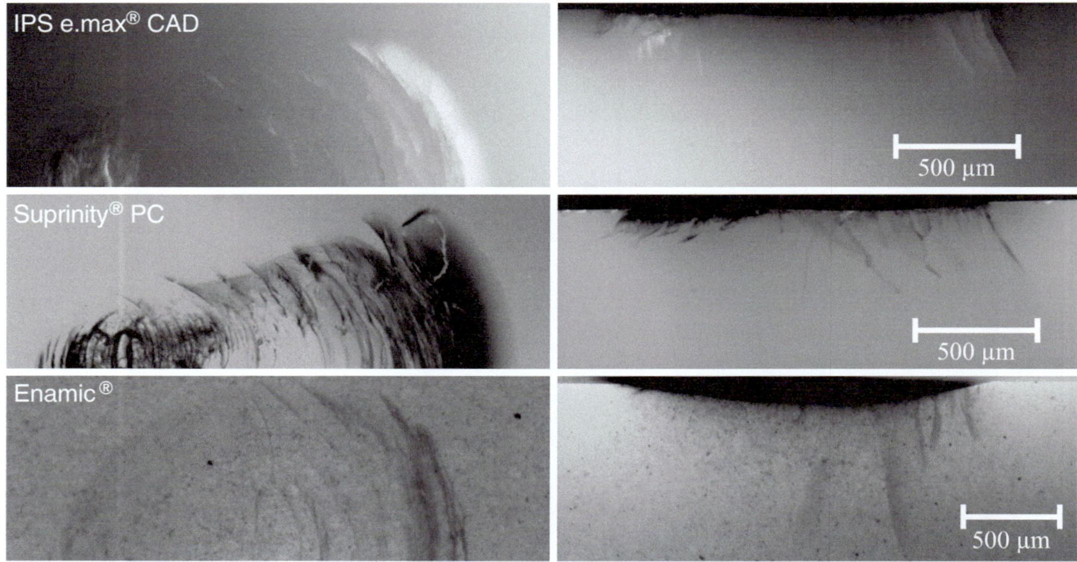

Fig. 3.16 Surface (left column) and subsurface (right column) damage on two lithium-based ceramics and one hybrid material after 10^4 cycles of frictional sliding contact loading with a spherical zirconia ball on a 30° tilted substrate at 200 N. Taken from Ref. [133]. Rreprinted with permission from Elsevier

phases, added to stress corrosion, the *degradation of toughening mechanisms* (responsible for R-curve effects) is the other main phenomenon reducing their lifetime during cyclic loading. This takes place in glass-ceramics and polycrystalline ceramics, where *crack bridging* is the main crack shielding mechanism. During repeated unloading and reloading, the friction between opposing crack faces is reduced, degrading frictional bridges: R-curves become thereby flatter with increasing number of cycles. This is called "*true fatigue effect*," in purely mechanical terms.

In materials having a marked R-curve due to bridging, cyclic crack growth da/dt can be modelled by the development and maturation of an equilibrium steady-state "cyclic R-curve," which can be partitioned into bridging degradation and accumulation rates, respectively as [134]:

$$\frac{\mathrm{d}a}{\mathrm{d}t} = \left(\frac{\partial K_{\mathrm{I,br}}}{\partial t}\right)\left(\frac{\partial K_{\mathrm{I,br}}}{\partial a}\right)^{-1}, \qquad (3.27)$$

with the $\partial K_{\mathrm{br}}/\partial a$ accumulation term being a strong function of K_{max} and determining the slope of the cyclic R-curve (which is less pronounced than an R-curve obtained from monotonic loading). A dependency on ΔK (and therefore on R-ratio) should be proportional to the crack opening displacement Δu, which is in turn directly proportional to the length of the fiber that is allowed to slide out of its socket. For random orientations with high aspect ratio particulates, the density function for interlocking events (rather than pull-out events) must be higher than for low aspect ratio particulates, limiting Δu and thus conserving K_{br}. This is especially the case for small cracks where the contribution of elastic bridges predominate at the beginning of the R-curve development [95].

The degradation of the $K_{\mathrm{I,br}}$ term can be used to indirectly derive the existence of crack bridging elements by combining crack growth rate measurements in static (or dynamic) and cyclic tests. In "bridging materials," the crack growth exponent n **must** differ for cracks that remain open during the entire crack growth range Δa ($a_{\mathrm{c}} - a_{\mathrm{i}}$)—such as in static or dynamic tests—and for cracks that are periodically (re)opened and (re)closed. This is based on the assumption that the $\sigma_{\mathrm{br,fr}}$ contribution is reduced with increasing number of cycles [93], as a direct result of the degradation of the initial coefficient of friction μ_i between the fiber and the matrix [135]:

$$\mu = \mu_i \exp\left(-N / N_0\right) \qquad (3.28)$$

with N_0 being a characteristic number of cycles. The lifetime t_f, therefore, should decrease for the cyclic condition relative to the static condition if bridging is a relevant toughening mechanism. The effect on the n-value is thus:

$$n_{\text{static}} = n_{\text{cyclic}} \frac{\sigma Y \sqrt{a'}}{\sigma Y \sqrt{a'} + K'_{\text{I,br}}} > n_{\text{cyclic}} \qquad (3.29)$$

being a' any crack size within $a_i < a' < a_c$ and $K'_{\text{br}} < 0$ [110]. Once $n_{\text{static}} > n_{\text{cyclic}}$ is established, one must assume the existence of an R-curve and that a "*true fatigue effect*" took place. Otherwise, that is, if no R-curve exists, the condition $n_{\text{static}} = n_{\text{cyclic}}$ must result, and n_{static} is the sole consequence of SCG. In R-curve materials (i.e., $n_{\text{static}} > n_{\text{cyclic}}$), SCG effects cannot be disentangled from R-curve effects in the subcritical regime; the n_{static} values of the same material with and without an R-curve, would rank $n_{\text{s,SCG}} < n_{\text{s,SCG + R-curve}}$. It follows from these concepts that lifetime predictions based on n_{static} values will be invariably overestimated for R-curve materials, or match to experimentally obtained cyclic lifetimes if no R-curve is existent.

Conversely to the effect of a low R-ratio, which is expected to accelerate the degradation of the friction stress that contributes to K_{br}, an increase in testing frequency hardly affects K_{br} in relevant frequencies for application, being experimentally detectable for increases in frequency by over 2 orders of magnitude, depending on material [136].

References

1. ISO 6872. Dentistry—ceramic materials. Geneva: International Organization for Standardization; 2015.
2. Jayatilaka ADS, Trustrum K. Statistical approach to brittle-fracture. J Mater Sci. 1977;12:1426–30.
3. Weibull W. A statistical distribution function of wide applicability. J Appl Mech. 1951;18:293–7.
4. Weibull W. A statistical theory of the strength of materials, Ingenlorsvetenakapademiens Handlinger. Stockholm: Generalstabens litografiska anstalts förlag; 1930.
5. EN-843-5. Mechanical testing of monolithic ceramics at room temperature. Part 5: Statistical treatment. 1997.
6. Danzer R, Supancic P, Pascual J, Lube T. Fracture statistics of ceramics—Weibull statistics and deviations from Weibull statistics. Eng Fract Mech. 2007;74:2919–32.
7. Lohbauer U, Belli R, Arnetzl G, Scherrer SS, Quinn G. Fracture of a veneered-ZrO2 dental prosthesis from an inner thermal crack. Case Stud Eng Fail Anal. 2014;2:100–6.
8. Belli R, Lohbauer U. The breakdown of the Weibull behavior in dental zirconias. J Am Ceram Soc. 2021;104:4819–28.
9. Belli R, Scherrer SS, Lohbauer U. Report on fractures of trilayered all-ceramic fixed dental prostheses. Case Stud Eng Fail Analysis. 2016;7:71–9.
10. Belli R, Volkl H, Csato S, Tremmel S, Wartzack S, Lohbauer U. Development of a hoop-strength test for model sphero-cylindrical dental ceramic crowns: FEA and fractography. J Eur Ceram Soc. 2020;40:4753–64.
11. Munz D, Fett T. Ceramics: mechanical properties, failure behavior, materials selection. Berlin: Springer; 1999.
12. Gorjan L, Ambrozic M. Bend strength of alumina ceramics: a comparison of Weibull statistics with other statistics based on very large experimental data set. J Eur Ceram Soc. 2012;32:1221–7.
13. Danzer R, Lube T, Supancic P. Monte Carlo simulations of strength distributions of brittle materials—type of distribution, specimen and sample size. Zeitschrift Fur Metallkunde. 2001;92:773–83.
14. Quinn GD. Weibull strength scaling for standardized rectangular flexure specimens. J Am Ceram Soc. 2003;86:508–10.
15. Wendler M, Belli R, Petschelt A, Mevec D, Harrer W, Lube T, et al. Chairside CAD/CAM materials. Part 2: flexural strength testing. Dent Mater. 2017;33:99–109.
16. Baratta FI, Matthews WT, Quinn GD. Errors associated with flexure testing of brittle materials. Report no. MTL TR 87–35, US Army Materials Technology Laboratory. 1987.
17. Quinn GD, Morell R. Design data for engineering ceramics: a review of the flexure test. J Am Ceram Soc. 1991;74:2037–66.
18. Lube T, Manner M, Danzer R. The miniaturization of the 4-point-bend test. Fatigue Fract Eng Mater Struct. 1997;30:1605–16.
19. Pick B, Meira JBC, Driemeier L, Braga RR. A critical view on biaxial and short-beam uniaxial flexural strength tests applied to resin composites using

Weibull, fractographic and finite element analysis. Dent Mater. 2010;26:83–90.

20. Lube T, Manner M. Development of a bending-test device for small samples. Key Eng Mater. 1997;132–136:488–91.

21. Belli R, Wendler M, Zorzin JI, Lohbauer U. Practical and theoretical considerations on the fracture toughness testing of dental restorative materials. Dent Mater. 2018;34:97–119.

22. Staudacher M, Lube T, Schlacher J, Supancic P. Comparison of biaxial strength measured with the ball-on-three-balls and the ring-on-ring-test. Open Ceram. 2021;6:100101.

23. Börger A, Supancic P, Danzer R. The ball on three balls test for strength testing of brittle discs: stress distribution in the disc. J Eur Ceram Soc. 2002;22:1425–36.

24. Börger A, Supancic P, Danzer R. The ball on three balls test for strength testing of brittle discs: part II: analysis of possible errors in the strength determination. J Eur Ceram Soc. 2004;24:2917–28.

25. Danzer R, Supancic P, Harrer W. Biaxial tensile strength test for brittle rectangular plates. J Ceram Soc Jpn. 2006;114:1054–60.

26. Harrer W, Danzer R, Supancic P, Lube T. The ball on three balls test: strength testing of specimens of different sizes and geometries. Proceedings of the 10th ECerS Conference. 2007. p. 1271–5.

27. Irwin GR. Analysis of stresses and strains near the end of a crack traversing a plate. J Appl Mech. 1957;24:361–4.

28. Inglis CE. Stresses in a plate due to the presence of cracks and sharp corners. Trans Inst Naval Archit. 1913;55:219–41.

29. Griffith AA. The phenomena of rupture and flow in solids. Phil Trans R Soc Lond A. 1921;221:168–98.

30. Wieghardt K. Über das Spalten und Zerreissen elastischer Körper. Z Math Phys. 1907;55:60–103.

31. Soderholm KJ. Review of the fracture toughness approach. Dent Mater. 2010;26:E63–77.

32. Danzer R. On the relationship between ceramic strength and the requirements for mechanical design. J Eur Ceram Soc. 2014;34:3435–60.

33. Quinn GD, Swab JJ. Fracture toughness of glasses as measured by the SCF and SEPB methods. J Eur Ceram Soc. 2017;37:4243–57.

34. Quinn GD, Swab JJ, Motyka MJ. Fracture toughness of a toughened silicon nitride by ASTM C 1421. J Am Ceram Soc. 2003;86:1043–5.

35. Quinn GD. Refinements to the surface crack in flexure method for fracture toughness of ceramics. J Eur Ceram Soc (Vii, Pt 1–3). 2002;206-2:633–6.

36. Quinn GD. The fracture toughness round robins in VAMAS: what we have learned. In: Salem JA, Quinn GD, Jenkins MG, editors. Fracture resistance testing of monolithic and composite brittle materials, ASTM STP 1409. West Conshohocken, PA: ASTM International; 2002. p. 107–26.

37. Quinn GD, Salem JA. Effect of lateral cracks on fracture toughness determined by the surface-crack-in-flexure method. J Am Ceram Soc. 2002;85:873–80.

38. Swab JJ, Quinn GD. Effect of precrack "halos" on fracture toughness determined by the surface crack in flexure method. J Am Ceram Soc. 1998;81:2261–8.

39. Quinn G. On the applicability of ASTM Standard C 1421 for fracture toughness KIc to glasses and dental restorative materials. Oral presentation at the ACerS Meeting, Daytona Beach. 2015.

40. Quinn GD, Gettings RJ, Kübler JJ. Fracture toughness of ceramics by the surface crack in flexure method: results from the VAMASround robin. Ceram Eng Sci Proc. 1994;15:846–55.

41. Quinn GD, Salem J, Baron I, Cho K, Foley M, Fang H. Fracture-toughness of advanced ceramics at room-temperature. J Res Natl Inst Stand Technol. 1992;97:579–607.

42. Anstis GR, Chantikul P, Lawn BR, Marshall DB. A critical-evaluation of indentation techniques for measuring fracture-toughness. 1. Direct crack measurements. J Am Ceram Soc. 1981;64:533–8.

43. Munz DG, Shannon JL, Bubsey RT. Fracture-toughness calculation from maximum load in 4 point bend tests of Chevron notch specimens. Int J Fract. 1980;16:R137–R41.

44. ASTM C1421. Standard test methods for determination of fracture toughness of advances ceramics at ambient temperature. West Conshohocken: ASTM International; 2010.

45. ISO18756. Fine ceramics (advanced ceramics, advanced technical ceramics)—determination of fracture toughness of monolithic ceramics at room temperature by the surface crack in flexure (SCF) method. Geneva: International Organization for Standardization; 2003.

46. ISO24370. Fine ceramics (advanced ceramics, advanced technical ceramics)—test method for fracture toughness of monolithic ceramics at room temperature by chevron-notched beam (CNB) method. Geneva: International Organization for Standardization; 2005.

47. ISO15732. Fine ceramics (advanced ceramics, advanced technical ceramics)—test method for fracture toughness of monolithic ceramics at room temperature by single edge precracked beam (SEPB) method. Geneva: International Organization for Standardization; 2003.

48. Marshall DB, Evans AG. Comment on elastic-plastic indentation damage in ceramics—the median-radial crack system—reply. J Am Ceram Soc. 1981;64:C182–C3.

49. Evans AG, Charles EA. Fracture toughness determinations by indentation. J Am Ceram Soc. 1976;59:371–2.

50. Chantikul P, Anstis GR, Lawn BR, Marshall DB. A critical-evaluation of indentation techniques for measuring fracture-toughness. 2. Strength method. J Am Ceram Soc. 1981;64:539–43.

51. Miyazaki H, Yoshizawa Y. A reinvestigation of the validity of the indentation fracture (IF) method as applied to ceramics. J Eur Ceram Soc. 2017;37:4437–41.

52. Miyazaki H, Yoshizawa Y. Correlation of the indentation fracture resistance measured using high-resolution optics and the fracture toughness obtained by the single edge-notched beam (SEPB) method for typical structural ceramics with various microstructures. Ceram Int. 2016;42:7873–6.

53. Quinn GD, Bradt RC. On the Vickers indentation fracture toughness test. J Am Ceram Soc. 2007;90:673–80.

54. Wang H, Isgro G, Pallav P, Feilzer AJ, Chao YL. Influence of test methods on fracture toughness of a dental porcelain and a soda lime glass. J Am Ceram Soc. 2005;88:2868–73.

55. Newman JC, Raju IS. An empirical stress-intensity factor equation for the surface crack. Eng Fract Mech. 1981;15:185–92.

56. Strobl S, Supancic P, Lube T, Danzer R. Corrigendum to "surface crack in tension or in bending—a reassessment of the Newman and Raju formula in respect to fracture toughness measurements in brittle materials (vol 32, pg 1491, 2012)". J Eur Ceram Soc. 2018;38:355–8.

57. Strobl S, Supancic P, Lube T, Danzer R. Surface crack in tension or in bending—a reassessment of the Newman and Raju formula in respect to fracture toughness measurements in brittle materials. J Eur Ceram Soc. 2012;32:1491–501.

58. Lube T, Rasche S, Nindhia TGT. A fracture toughness test using the ball-on-three-balls test. J Am Ceram Soc. 2016;99:249–56.

59. Belli R, Wendler M, Petschelt A, Lube T, Lohbauer U. Fracture toughness testing of biomedical ceramic-based materials using beams, plates and discs. J Eur Ceram Soc. 2018;38:5533–44.

60. Fett T. Influence of a finite notch root radius on fracture toughness. J Eur Ceram Soc. 2005;25:543–7.

61. Kübler J. Fracture toughness using the SEVNB method: preliminary results. Ceram Eng Sci Proc. 1997;18:155–62.

62. Turon-Vinas M, Anglada M. Fracture toughness of zirconia from a shallow notch produced by ultra-short pulsed laser ablation. J Eur Ceram Soc. 2014;34:3865–70.

63. Turon-Vinas M, Anglada M. Assessment in Si3N4 of a new method for determining the fracture toughness from a surface notch micro-machined by ultra-short pulsed laser ablation. J Eur Ceram Soc. 2015;35:1737–41.

64. Carlton HD, Elmer JW, Freeman DC, Schaeffer RD, Derkach O, Gallegos GF. Laser notching ceramics for reliable fracture toughness testing. J Eur Ceram Soc. 2016;36:227–34.

65. Zhao W, Rao PG, Ling ZY. A new method for the preparation of ultra-sharp V-notches to measure fracture toughness in ceramics. J Eur Ceram Soc. 2014;34:4059–62.

66. Belli R, Zorzin JI, Lohbauer U. Fracture toughness testing of dental materials: a critical evaluation. Curr Oral Health Rep. 2018;5:163–8.

67. Bajaj D, Arola DD. On the R-curve behavior of human tooth enamel. Biomaterials. 2009;30:4037–46.

68. Evans AG. Perspectives on the development of high-toughness ceramics. J Am Ceram Soc. 1990;73:187.

69. Evans AG, Cannon RM. Toughening of brittle solids by martensitic transformations. Acta Metall. 1986;34:761–800.

70. Evans AG, Mcmeeking RM. On the toughening of ceramics by strong reinforcements. Acta Metall. 1986;34:2435–41.

71. Evans AG, Heuer AH. Transformation toughening and its role in structural ceramic design. J Miner Met Mater Soc. 1982;35:A32.

72. Mcmeeking RM, Evans AG. Mechanics of transformation-toughening in brittle materials. J Am Ceram Soc. 1982;65:242–6.

73. Evans AG, Faber KT. Toughening of ceramics by circumferential microcracking. J Am Ceram Soc. 1981;64:394–8.

74. Fünfschilling S, Fett T, Hoffmann J, Oberacker R, Özcoban H, Schneider GA, et al. Estimation of the high-temperature R-curve for ceramics from strength measurements including specimens with focused ion beam notches. J Am Ceram Soc. 2010;93:2411–4.

75. Fett T, Munz D. R-curve for a lead zirconate titanate ceramic obtained from tensile strength tests with Knoop-damaged specimens. J Am Ceram Soc. 2000;83:3199–201.

76. Munz D. What can we learn from R-curve measurements? J Am Ceram Soc. 2007;90:1–15.

77. Burghard Z, Zimmermann A, Rodel J, Aldinger F, Lawn BR. Crack opening profiles of indentation cracks in normal and anomalous glasses. Acta Mater. 2004;52:293–7.

78. Fett T, Munz D, Kounga Njiwa AB, Rödel J, Quinn GD. Bridging stresses in sintered reaction-bonded Si_3N_4 from COD measurements. J Eur Ceram Soc. 2005;25:29–36.

79. Rödel J, Kelly JF, Lawn BR. In situ measurements of bridged crack interfaces in the scanning electron microscope. J Am Ceram Soc. 1990;73:3313–8.

80. Seidel J, Rödel J. Measurement of crack tip toughness in alumina as a function of grain size. J Am Ceram Soc. 1997;80:433–8.

81. Deubener J, Höland M, Höland W, Janakiraman N, Rheinberger VM. Crack tip fracture toughness of base glasses for dental restoration glass-ceramics using crack opening displacements. J Mech Behav Biomed Mater. 2011;4:1291–8.

82. Knehans R, Steinbrech R. Memory effects of crack resistance during slow crack growth in notched Al2O3 bend specimens. J Mater Sci Lett. 1982;1:327–9.

83. Fett T, Funfschilling S, Hoffmann MJ, Oberacker R. Different R-curves for two- and three-dimensional cracks. Int J Fract. 2008;153:153–9.

84. Marschall DB, Swain MV. Crack resistance curves in magnesia-partially-stabilized zirconia. J Am Ceram Soc. 1988;71:399–407.

85. Steinbrech R, Schmenkel O. Crack resistance curves for surface cracks in alumina. J Am Ceram Soc. 1988;71:C-271–3.

86. Steinbrech RW, Reichl A, Schaarwachter W. R-curve behavior of long cracks in alumina. J Am Ceram Soc. 1990;73:2009–15.

87. Kruzic JJ, Satet RL, Hoffmann MJ, Cannon RM, Ritchie RO. The utility of R-curves for understanding fracture toughness-strength relations in bridging ceramics. J Am Ceram Soc. 2008;91:1986–94.

88. Funfschilling S, Fett T, Hoffmann MJ, Oberacker R, Schwind T, Wippler J, et al. Mechanisms of toughening in silicon nitrides: the roles of crack bridging and microstructure. Acta Mater. 2011;59:3978–89.

89. Belli R, Wendler M, Cicconi MR, de Ligny D, Petschelt A, Werbach K, et al. Fracture anisotropy in texturized lithium disilicate glass-ceramics. J Non-Cryst Solids. 2018;481:457–69.

90. Wendler M, Belli R, Schachtner M, Amberger G, Petschelt A, Fey T, et al. Resistance curves of short-fiber reinforced methacrylate-based biomedical composites. Eng Fract Mech. 2018;190:146–58.

91. Tiu J, Belli R, Lohbauer U. Rising R-curves in particulate/fiber-reinforced resin composite layered systems. J Mech Behav Biomed Mater. 2019;103:103537.

92. Foulk-III JW, Johnson GC, Klein PA, Ritchie RO. On the toughening of brittle materials by grain bridging: promoting intergranular fracture through grain angle, strength and toughness. J Mech Phys Solids. 2008;56:2381–400.

93. Fett T. New contributions to R-curves and bridging stresses—applications of weight functions. Karlsruhe: KIT Scientific; 2012.

94. Foulk JW, Cannon RM, Johnson GC, Klein PA, Ritchie RO. A micromechanical basis for partitioning the evolution of grain bridging in brittle materials. J Mech Phys Solids. 2007;55:719–43.

95. Gallops S, Fett T, Kruzic JJ. Fatigue threshold R-curve behavior of grain bridging ceramics: role of grain size and grain-boundary adhesion. J Am Ceram Soc. 2011;94:2556–61.

96. Kirsten J, Belli R, Wendler M, Petschelt A, Hurle K, Lohbauer U. Crack growth rates in lithium disilicates with bulk (mis)alignment of the Li2Si2O5 phase in the [001] direction. J Non-Cryst Solids. 2020;532:119877.

97. Quinn JB, Sundar V, Lloyd IK. Influence of microstructure and chemistry on the fracture toughness of dental ceramics. Dent Mater. 2003;19:603–11.

98. Faber KT, Evans AG. 2 toughening mechanisms—crack deflection and microcracking. Am Ceram Soc Bull. 1981;60:382.

99. Casellas D, Cumbrera FL, Sanchez-Bajo F, Forsling W, Llanes L, Anglada M. On the transformation toughening of Y-ZrO2 ceramics with mixed Y-TZP/PSZ microstructures. J Eur Ceram Soc. 2001;21:765–77.

100. Bechtle S, Fett T, Rizzi G, Habelitz S, Schneider G. Mixed-mode stress intensity factors for kink cracks with finite kink length loaded in tension and in bending: application to dentin and enamel. J Mech Behav Biomed Mater. 2010;3:303–12.

101. Bechtle S, Habelitz S, Klocke A, Fett T, Schneider G. The fracture behaviour of dental enamel. Biomaterials. 2010;31:375–84.

102. Bechtle S, Fett T, Rizzi G, Habelitz S, Klocke A, Schneider GA. Crack arrest within teeth at the dentinoenamel junction caused by elastic modulus mismatch. Biomaterials. 2010;31:4238–47.

103. Bajaj D, Arola D. Role of prism decussation on fatigue crack growth and fracture of human enamel. Acta Biomater. 2009;5:3045–56.

104. Gonzaga CC, Okada CY, Cesar PF, Miranda WG Jr, Yoshimura HN. Effect of processing induced particle alignment on the fracture toughness and fracture behavior of multiphase dental ceramics. Dent Mater. 2009;25:1293–301.

105. Belli R, Wendler M, Petschelt A, Lohbauer U. Mixed-mode fracture toughness of texturized LS2 glass-ceramics using the three-point bending with eccentric notch test. Dent Mater. 2017;33:1473–7.

106. Freiman SW, Wiederhorn SM, J. MJJ. Environmentally enhanced fracture of glass: a historical perspective. J Am Ceram Soc. 2009;92:1371–82.

107. Michalske TA, Freiman SW. A molecular mechanism for stress corrosion in vitreous silica. J Am Ceram Soc. 1983;66:284–8.

108. Wiederhorn SM, Bolz LH. Stress corrosion and static fatigue of glass. J Am Ceram Soc. 1970;53:543–8.

109. Wiederhorn SM. Influence of water vapor on crack propagation in soda-lime glass. J Am Ceram Soc. 1967;50:407–14.

110. Munz D, Fett T. Ceramics. Berlin: Springer; 2001.

111. Wendler M, Belli R, Valladares D, Petschelt A, Lohbauer U. Chairside CAD/CAM materials. Part 3: cyclic fatigue parameters and lifetime predictions. Dent Mater. 2018;34:910–21.

112. Borba M, de Araújo MD, Fukushima KA, Yoshimura HN, Cesar PF, Griggs JA, et al. Effect of the microstructure on the lifetime of dental ceramics. Dent Mater. 2011;27:710–21.

113. Teixeira EC, Piascik JR, Stoner BR, Thompson JY. Dynamic fatigue and strength characterization of three ceramic materials. J Mater Sci Mater Med. 2007;18:1219–24.

114. Mitov G, Gessner J, Lohbauer U, Woll K, Muecklich F, Pospiech P. Subcritical crack growth behavior and life data analysis of two types of dental Y-TZP. Dent Mater. 2011;27:684–91.

115. Zhang F, Reveron H, Spies BC, Van Meerbeek B, Chevalier J. Trade-off between fracture resistance and translucency of zirconia and lithium-disilicate glass ceramics for monolithic restorations. Acta Biomater. 2019;91:24–34.

116. Griggs JA, Alaqeel SM, Zhang Y, Miller AW III, Cai Z. Effects of stress rate and calculation method on the subcritical crack growth parameters deduced from constant stress-rate flexural testing. Dent Mater. 2011;27:364–70.

117. Gonzaga CC, Cesar PF, Miranda WG Jr, Yoshimura HN. Slow crack growth and reliability of dental ceramics. Dent Mater. 2011;27:394–406.
118. Lohbauer U, Petschelt A, Greil P. Lifetime prediction of CAD/CAM dental ceramics. J Biomed Mater Res. 2002;63:780–5.
119. Ramos NC, Campos TMB, de La Paz IS, Machado JPB, Bottino MA, Cesar PF, et al. Microstructure characterization and SCG of newly engineered dental ceramics. Dent Mater. 2016;32:870–8.
120. Joshi GV, Duan Y, Della Bona A, Hill T, St. John K, Griggs JA. Contributions of stress corrosion and cyclic fatigue to subcritical crack growth in a dental glass-ceramic. Dent Mater. 2014;30:884–90.
121. Belli R, Zorzin JI, Petschelt A, Lohbauer U, Rocca GT. Crack growth behavior of a biomedical polymer-ceramic interpenetrating scaffolds composite in the subcritical regimen. Eng Fract Mech. 2020;231:107014.
122. Barlet M, Delaye JM, Boizot B, Bonamy D, Caraballo R, Peuget S, et al. From network depolymerization to stress corrosion cracking in sodium-borosilicate glasses: effect of the chemical composition. J Non-Cryst Solids. 2016;450:174–84.
123. Belli R, Wendler M, Zorzin JI, Petschelt A, Tanaka CB, Meira J, et al. Descriptions of crack growth behaviors in glass-ZrO2 bilayers under thermal residual stresses. Dent Mater. 2016;32:1165–76.
124. Pinto MM, Cesar PF, Rosa V, Yoshimura HN. Influence of slow crack growth of dental porcelains. Dent Mater. 2008;24:814–23.
125. Charles RJ. Dynamic fatigue of glass. J Appl Phys. 1958;29:1657–61.
126. Fett T, Martin G, Munz D, Thun G. Determination of d a/d N-ΔK1 curves for small cracks in alumina in alternating bending tests. J Mater Sci. 1991;26:3320–8.
127. Thoman DR, Bain LJ, Antle CE. Inferences on the parameters of the Weibull distribution. Technometrics. 1969;11:445–60.
128. Evans AG, Fuller ER. Crack-propagation in ceramic materials under cyclic loading conditions. Metall Mater Trans B. 1974;5:27–33.
129. Lawn BR. Partial cone crack formation in a brittle material loaded with a sliding spherical indenter. Proc R Soc Lond. 1967;299:307–16.
130. Ren LL, Zhang Y. Sliding contact fracture of dental ceramics: principles and validation. Acta Biomater. 2014;10:3243–53.
131. Chai H. Multi-crack analysis of hydraulically pumped cone fracture in brittle solids under cyclic spherical contact. Int J Fract. 2007;143:1–14.
132. Zhang Y, Sailer I, Lawn BR. Fatigue of dental ceramics. J Dent. 2013;41:1135–47.
133. Wendler M, Kaizer MR, Belli R, Lohbauer U, Zhang Y. Sliding contact wear and subsurface damage of CAD/CAM materials against zirconia. Dental Mater. 2020;36(3):387–401.
134. Jacobs DS, Chen IW. Cyclic fatigue in ceramics—a balance between crack shielding accumulation and degradation. J Am Ceram Soc. 1995;78:513–20.
135. Fett T, Kraft O, Munz D. Fatigue failure of coarse-grained alumina under contact loading. Mater Werkst. 2005;26:163–70.
136. Fett T, Munz D. Differences between static and cyclic fatigue effects in alumina. J Mater Sci Lett. 1993;12:352–4.

We might start asking ourselves the meaning behind concepts like "forensic & structural determination" or "fractographic analysis"? Figure 4.1 shows us the complementary duality of destruction and construction. In order to teach a proper construction design and to derive certain preparation guidelines, we first need to learn from our deficiencies. We need to study clinical failures, connect them to the individual material performance and need to identify substantial reasons for failure. A typical fractographic procedure is a meticulous collection of any details involved in the history of the target restoration, the structural features of the used material, and the observation of the fracture planes in order to derive guiding conclusions.

In general, a fractographic procedure (according to EN 843-6) consists of:

- Objection (status quo, history, procedures, materials, environment, etc.)
- Action (collection, preparation, inspection, optical, chemical, structural analysis).
- Deduction (fracture features, cause and origin of failure, circumstances, classification).
- Result (presentation, conclusions, guidance).

Such standard operating procedures (SOPs) are commonly recommended in international standards, as there are the EN 843-6:2009 standard (Advanced technical ceramics—Mechanical properties of monolithic ceramics at room temperature—Part 6: Guidance for fractographic investigation) [1] and the ASTM standard 1322-15 (Standard Practice for Fractography and Characterization of Fracture Origins in Advanced Ceramics) [2]. A broad reference guide, a comprehensive selection of publications and case studies, and any further reading can be found at: www.fractography.org.

The above SOP makes clear that a sound fractographic analysis is not just a simple image of a fractured surface, but rather a whole story to be complementary—forensically—collected. By diving into the field of fractography, it becomes suddenly evident that the validity of the analysis very much relies on the available information and history of the specific case. No specific skills or cutting-edge research equipment is actually needed for a sound fractographic examination, but rather careful inspections of the fracture plane, meticulous collection of details and understanding around the fracture event, and finally a high portion of patience!

4.1 Destruction: Experimental Proof and Clinical Reality

Brittle failure of a structural element is commonly expressed as spontaneous fracture, thereby creating two new surfaces—the corresponding fracture planes. Both parts offer identical patterns and match their inverted morphologies. We learned, the fracture process itself has a starting point—a critical flaw under

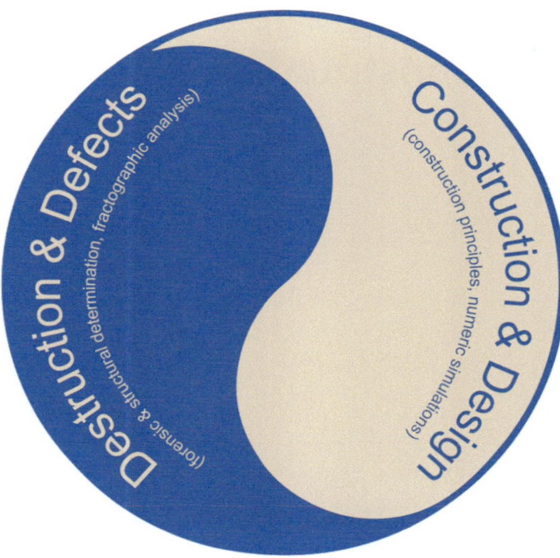

Fig. 4.1 Yin and Yang in construction design

maximum load—and an end point, characterized by compressive deflection of the fracture plane. Like in all kinetic processes, the velocity of this event is composed of an initial acceleration up to a maximum terminal velocity, related to the speed of sound in a material. This value is reported to reach 700–2500 m/s in glasses and to become even faster in ceramics [3]. As Griffith already back in 1921 postulated that cracks will grow when the elastically stored energy G, released by a brittle structure becomes greater than the increase in energy γ necessary for the formation of two new surfaces [4]:

$$G > 2\gamma \tag{4.1}$$

The terminal velocity is strongly depending on the speed of elastic waves (longitudinal elastic wave), the density, and the elastic constants (elastic modulus and Poisson ratio) of a material. The direction of crack propagation, however, is depending on the applied maximum tensile stress and structural irregularities arising from microstructural features and defect population. Therefore, the radial propagation of a crack front in a material is compromised by local deviations at varying velocities. Those disturbances of the crack front will be imprinted in a fractured surface and express themselves as readable fractographic patterns.

4.1.1　Examples: Lab Versus Clinical

The aspect of applied maximum tensile stress is an issue that might become extremely complicated in clinical reality. Stress states are not purely tensile in nature and in most cases superimposed by shear, bending, or compressive components. As the main practical consequence, the fractographic analysis of clinically failed specimens becomes much more complex and difficult, compared to the analysis of standardized, experimental test specimens. Figure 4.2 shows examples from either a standardized bending experiment or a clinically chipped molar crown. The fracture event in Fig. 4.2a is easy to trace as the starting point/fracture origin is characterized by the smooth fracture mirror, radial propagation, and mist and hackle regions. The end point is found on the opposite side of the specimen, leaving a compression curl, typical for bending experiments.

However, the clinical fracture event in Fig. 4.2b is more complex to analyze. The fracture origin is not clear to identify as the crack initiation is a result of repetitive fatigue, followed by wear and damage accumulation at the occlusal surface. A slight compression curl is observable, but the overall stress state remains unclear. In such cases, the history, occlusal contact situation, and opposing materials play a decisive role and need to be carefully collected from the dental technician, the dentist, and finally from the patient.

4.2　Fractography as a Bridging Tool

The definition of fractography appears rather general: "Fractography—means and methods for characterizing fractured specimens or components" [2] or lately modified to read as "Fractography—the field of study of fractures in materials, components and structures" [5].

Indeed, the idea of a forensic interpretation of fractured surfaces started with mainly observational, microscopic techniques. Over the years, this basic tool has been further developed,

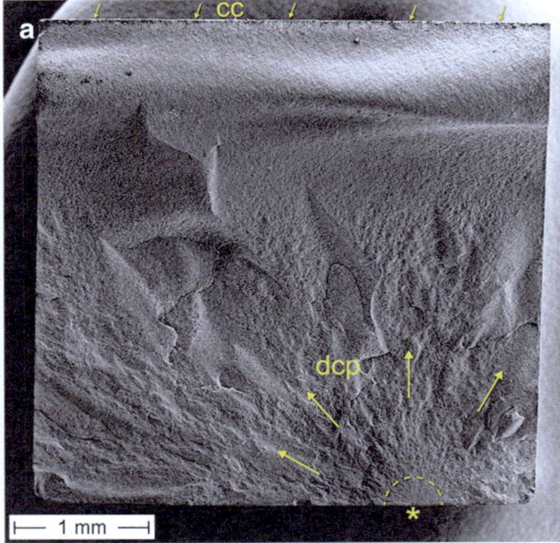

Fig. 4.2 Typical examples of fracture planes taken from (**a**) a fractured lithiumsilicate glass-ceramic specimen, fractured under 4-point bending load; and (**b**) a clinically fractured, molar implant-supported crown on tooth #27, exhibiting a veneer chipping on a zirconia substructure. The fracture origins (asterisks) are indicated as well as the direction of crack propagation (dcp) and the compression curl (cc)

specific and individual markings have been described, correlations to microstructural features have been derived, chemical or structural analytical methods have served as supportive tools, and finally three dimensional and quantitative fractography has entered the field in combination with fracture mechanics principles, making this tool today a unique scientific profession.

4.2.1   A Brief Introduction to Fractographic Methods

The most comprehensive and updated guide to fractographic techniques on brittle surfaces is the textbook written by George Quinn and published at NIST (free to download) [5]. Therein, one would find all types of techniques, microscopic equipment, specimen maintenance, analysis and interpretation of fractographic markings and further associated fields of contemporary research. All aspects therein are illustrated by fractographic examples from a wide range of applications, including clinical dentistry.

4.2.2   Fractography of Lab Specimens

The inspection of experimentally fractured specimens is a mandatory step supplementing the actual experiment. In most cases, fractures are intentionally created on standardized laboratory specimens approaching the strength or toughness properties of materials. Taking the example of measuring strength of a ceramic material, this procedure is described in the European Standard EN 843-1 [6]. The fractographic analysis is connected and described in EN 843-6 [1]. Based on a population of at least 30 specimens for a proper strength measurement, one should further investigate—beyond a certain strength value—on the reasons for failure and the inevitable implications on the scatter and distribution of data as brittle failure might originate from surface, edge or internal defects due to material inhomogeneities or processing flaws [7, 8]. Figure 4.3 illustrates the dependency of strength of a dental lithiumdisilicate ceramic on flaw type. The plot further shows the operator-dependent influence on fracture origin identification.

Figure 4.3 clearly shows that the operator has a prominent influence on the result, especially when analyzing difficult microstructures, such as fine-grained lithiumdisilicate glass-ceramics. One could further read from this plot, that surface defects are the prominent reason for failure in both, ground and polished groups. Surface defects are more clustered at higher strength in the polished group while comparably equally distributed over the whole strength range in the ground group. Pores play a minor role in both groups while edge defects might be more often detected in the ground group. Overall, the polishing procedure had a twofold effect, increasing on the one side the fracture strength from $\sigma_0 = 207$ MPa to $\sigma_0 = 276$ MPa (for this particular experimental 4-point bending setup) and elevating on the other side the Weibull modulus from $m = 7.9$ to $m = 9.3$.

The supplementary fractographic examination of fractured datasets is providing much insight toward the underlying fracture mecha-nisms. A bending test, however, is a comparably easy-to-interpret example. Once it comes to more complex stress states, even the fractographic examination becomes more difficult. A widely used alternative approach to strength is the biaxial testing of plates or discs [9]. The simplest and most obvious approach to those datasets might be counting the broken pieces and correlating them to the individual strength level [10]. Figure 4.4 shows such a collection of broken pieces for a single biaxial test of a dental ceramic material. Figure 4.5 further displays the number of broken pieces for two lithiumsilicate materials related to the measured biaxial strengths data.

Both materials in Fig. 4.5 are composed of similar glass-ceramic microstructure and offer comparable elastic constants [11]. By translating the number of broken pieces into actually, newly created surface area during fracture (and thus the energy release rate G), the Griffith fracture criterion:

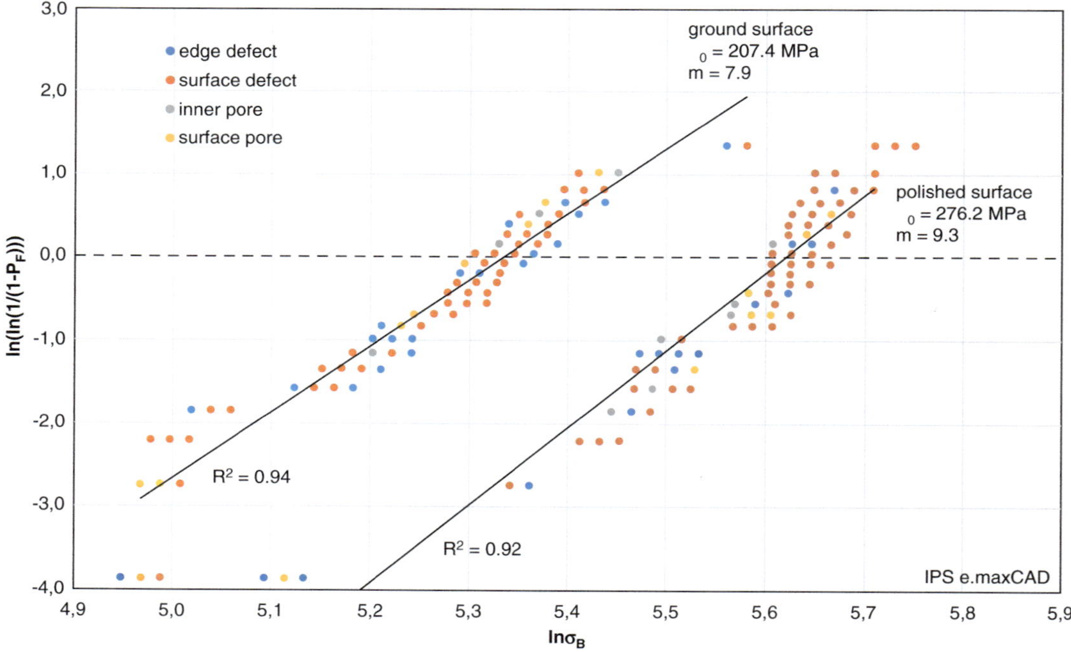

Fig. 4.3 Weibull plot of two strength datasets representing a ground versus a polished surface state of a lithium-disilicate glass-ceramic (IPS e.maxCAD, Ivoclar). Each strength data point has assigned three independent fracto-graphic assessments from trained operators. The fracture origins were assigned using a stereomicroscope under 20× magnification. Those data points showing four independent assessments were further analyzed using an SEM

$$\sigma_c = \sqrt{\frac{GE}{\pi a_c}} \qquad (4.2)$$

will explain that the number of broken pieces might work as a rough estimate for defect size a_c and with $K_{Ic} = GE$ also for the fracture toughness. According to Fig. 4.5, the material IPS e.max-CAD should offer a greater fracture toughness compared to the material Celtra Duo. Cross-referencing with literature data supports this observation as a K_{Ic} = 1.92–2.29 MPam$^{0.5}$ was measured for IPS e.maxCAD and a K_{Ic} = 1.52–1.68 MPam$^{0.5}$ for Celtra Duo [12]. Simple investigations on fractured biaxial discs might be further intensified by analysis of branching angles or analysis of the stress ratio distribution between σ_x and σ_y directions.

The actual fractographic examination of biaxial fracture origins, however, remains complicated, as a microscopic evaluation of all broken pieces seems unavoidable. At least, the region of maximum tensile stress is much smaller and concentrated at the center of a biaxial disc [9], so the search can be narrowed down to this region. In most cases, the fracture origin can be identified at the central part of the largest fragment. Morrell has published a useful practice guide on fractography of biaxial discs [13]. As disc fractures produce multiple fragments (see Fig. 4.4) which heavily complicate an optical inspection, this guide provides useful tutorials for the fractographic examination spanning from the general use of an adhesive tape on the compressive disc side to preserve the fragment arrangement up to the identification of the primary fracture origin via forking patterns.

4.2.2.1 Principal Fracture Markings

The fracture plane created by separating a specimen or a structural component into two pieces is always unique and individual for a given material, design, and stress state. In case of a pure elastic fracture, as expected for ceramic materials, both fracture planes offer identical topography. The identification of typical fracture patterns is the key to the interpretation of the fracture event.

As every individual fracture has a start and end point, the fracture origin and compression curl are in central focus of the analysis. In most cases, a trained fractographer would search for the compression curl first and trace back to the fracture origin by meticulously collecting fracture patterns along the crack path. Typical examples of compression curls are shown in Fig. 4.2. Compression curls are the result of a fracture in bending, where initial tensile stresses are transferred into compressive stresses at the end of a fracture event. A crack is always propagating along the easiest, least energy consuming, path through a material, finally entering a compressive zone and thus forming a curl pattern.

On the fracture plane, further patterns can be identified, all indicating the direction of crack propagation (dcp). Those patterns—next to the compression curl and fracture origin—typically

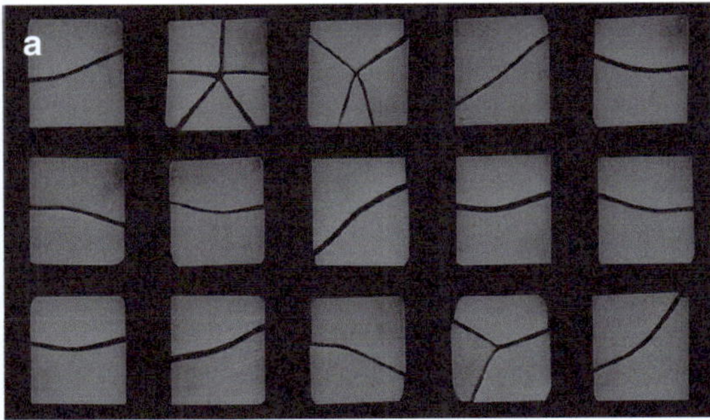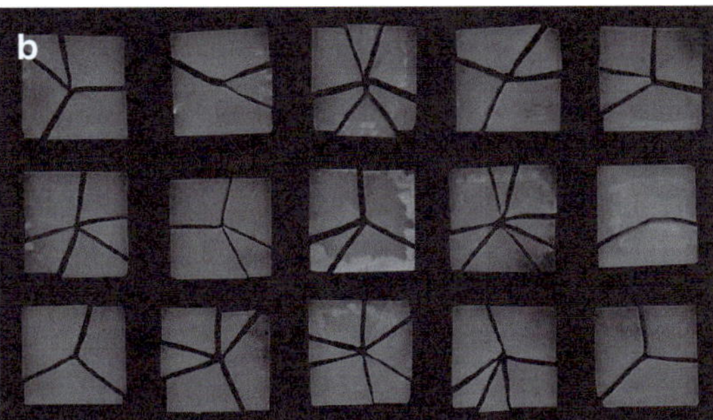

Fig. 4.4 Photograph of the reconstructed collection of broken fragments from a biaxial strength test for the material Celtra Duo (Dentsply): (**a**) coarse grinding with a red-labelled diamond bur and (**b**) fine polishing with a white-labelled diamond bur and subsequent polishing

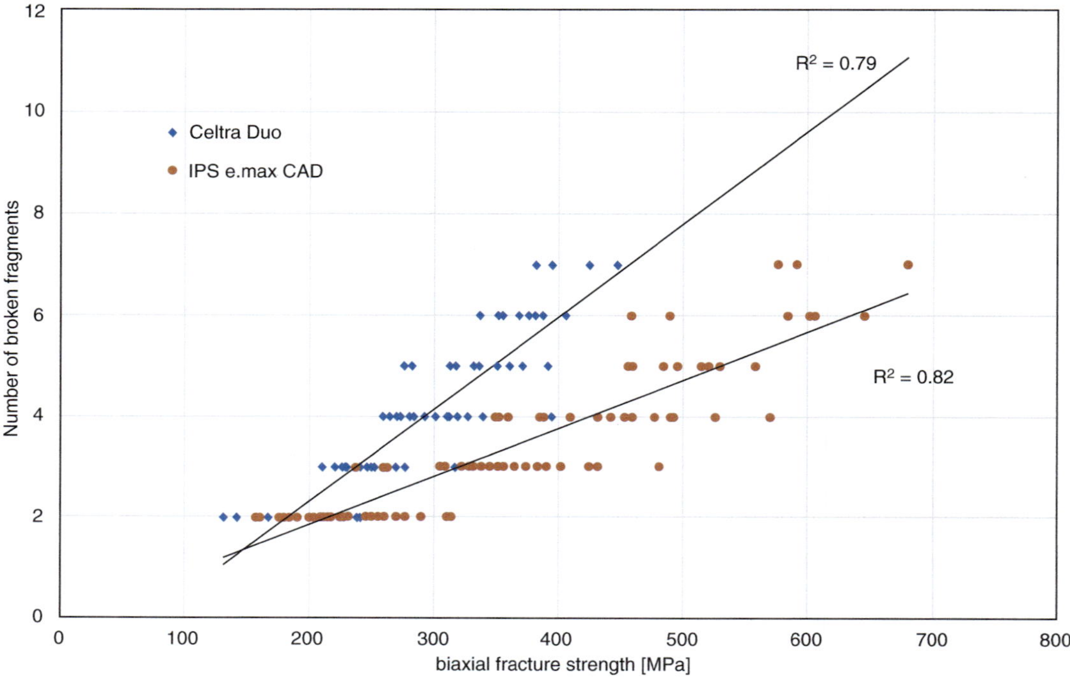

Fig. 4.5 Graphical analysis of number of broken pieces from biaxial strength testing related to the resulting biaxial strength data. A fair linear correlation at $r^2 = 0.79/0.82$ was achieved

include hackle (twist, wake) lines, arrest lines, Wallner lines, or even more specific features such as gull wings, internal defects (pores, inclusions), or edge chips. A detailed description of each fracture pattern would certainly exceed the scope of this chapter, but further reading is deeply recommended [5, 8]. Figure 4.6 shows examples of the most prominent patterns, typically found on brittle ceramic surfaces.

Finally, the fracture origin is of importance not simply indicating the starting point of a catastrophic failure, but more important as the source providing the actual reason for failure. Figure 4.7 shows a scheme of an ideal fracture origin surrounded by mirror, mist, and hackle regions, with increasing crack velocity.

The crack velocity is thereby determining the roughness of the morphology. At initial crack initiation (at the threshold toughness K_{I0}) a crack slowly increases velocity through the mirror region reaching its terminal velocity (at the fracture toughness K_{Ic}) in the mist and hackle region. Figure 4.8 illustrates the correlation of crack

velocity with fractographic fracture patterns in a model glass.

The knowledge of the fracture releasing defect size is of central importance in evaluating the underlying reason for failure. As the fracture strength σ_c is proportional to the inverse square root of the critical defect size a_c [see Eq. (4.2)], Fig. 4.9 schematically illustrates the various contributions to a defect population applied in glass engineering.

It is obvious to understand that the smaller the fracture releasing defect, the higher the resulting strength is expected. While defects based on fabrication might overlay the smaller microstructural defects, the damage resulting after a certain time in service might even further reduce the inherent strength of a material. The smaller unit of defect sizes are found in the microstructural scale, assuming that a defect-free, theoretical microstructure will practically not exist. The loading influence in service has a deleterious effect on all length scales, as described in crack growth and fatigue studies [15–17]. The

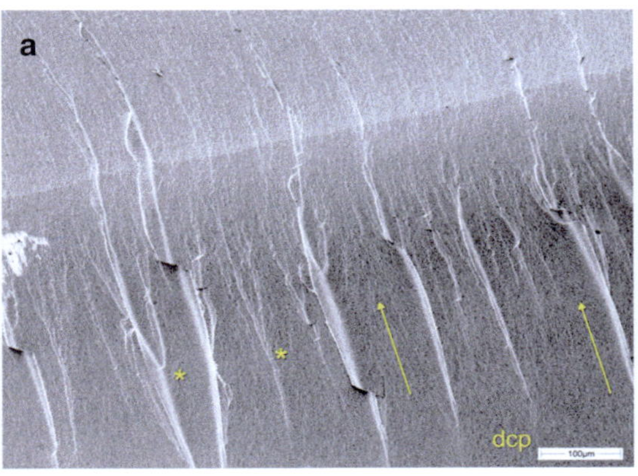
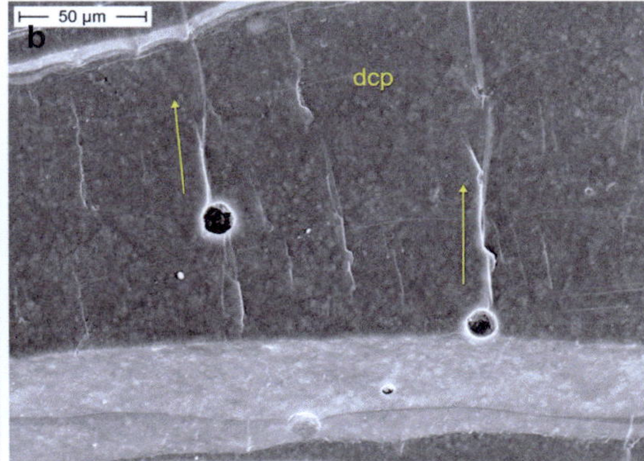

Fig. 4.6 Hackle lines are typical fracture markings indicating the dcp: (**a**) hackle, twist hackle (asterisks), and (**b**) wake hackle lines. Hackle lines are footprints of inclinations on the fracture plane and are best viewed under lateral illumination under a light microscope or under a SEM (as shown here)

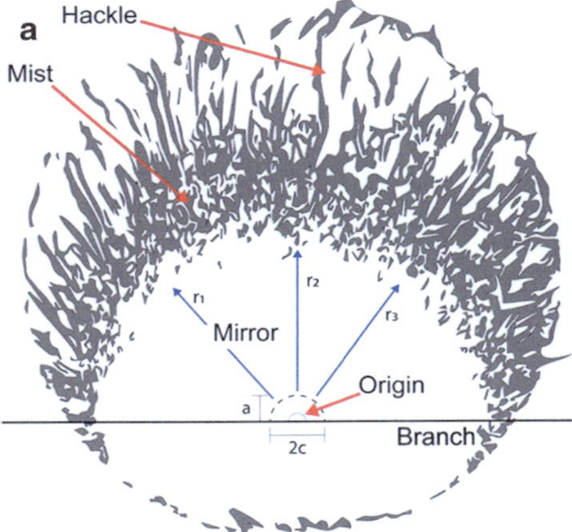
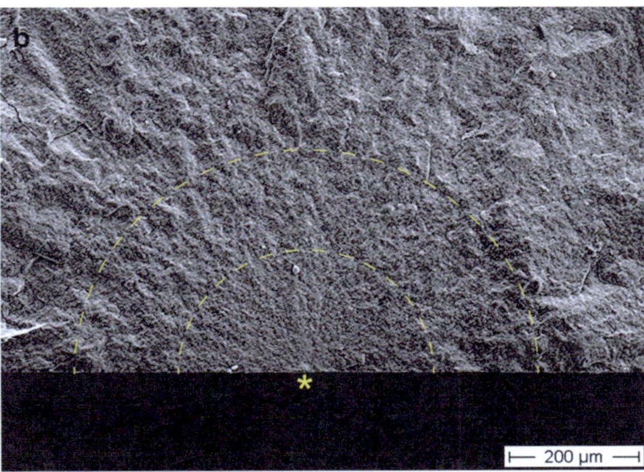

Fig. 4.7 Fracture origin on a brittle surface: (**a**) scheme indicating the three major regions—mirror, mist, and hackle, radially emanating from the fracture origin and (**b**) less prominent distinction between the regions on a glass-ceramic (dotted circles, two options; asterisk indicate fracture origin), microstructurally textured fracture surface. The region below the branch will stand for an internal flaw equally progressing in all directions

subcritical growth of a fracture releasing defect up to a critical diameter is indicated by the dotted line in Fig. 4.7.

Those rather general relations are commonly described for glass structures. In our dental ceramics, we are dealing with a more complicated, inhomogeneous microstructure. Based on Fig. 4.9, it becomes evident that in order to increase the performance of a brittle material, one approach is toward reduction of the maximum defect size via tailoring the microstructure and improving the surface quality, or by impeding or retarding the crack growth, thereby increasing the fracture toughness or introducing residual compressive stresses to a microstructure [14].

Tailoring the microstructure of a ceramic material (and hence enhancing the fracture toughness) is a key development approach to material improvement. All our dental ceramics are modified with second phase reinforcements in order to exhibit superior fracture resistance compared to pure, amorphous glass. Such reinforcements might be crystalline particles in an amorphous glass matrix

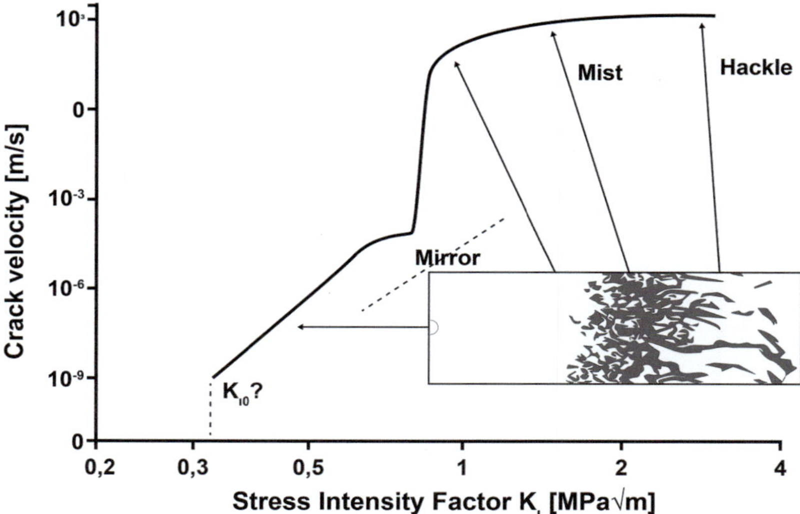

Fig. 4.8 Plot showing the relation of crack velocity v and the stress intensity K_I at the stage of crack initiation (v-K_I diagram, acc. to Bradt [14])

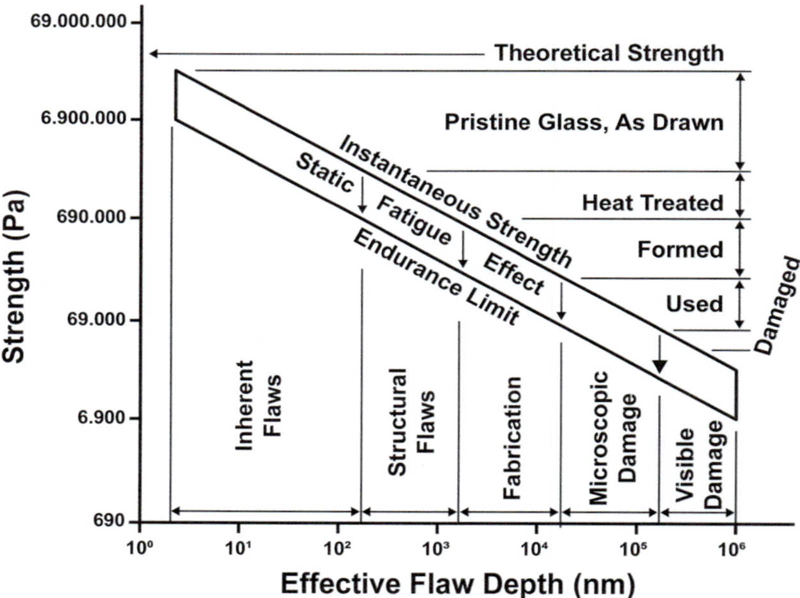

Fig. 4.9 Schematic contributions of different stages through glass production, treatment, and service to the defect population in glass and relation the expectable strength (acc. to Bradt [14])

(like in highly translucent veneering glasses), growth of a second crystalline phase at the expense of the amorphous glass phase (typically via the glass-ceramics process), or even glass-free, polycrystalline ceramics (such as our polycrystalline zirconia materials). With increasing fraction and size of the reinforcing phase, the fractographic distinctiveness of fracture patterns will diminish and the analysis will become more difficult.

Due to the fact, that a propagating crack will seek the easiest path through a material, new fracture features might arise from different microstructural morphologies. Figure 4.10 shows examples for a reinforced veneering glass (<20 vol% reinforcing phases of <15 μm mean crystallite size), a glass-ceramic (approx. 50 vol% reinforcing phase, of 1–2 μm mean crystallite sizes), and a polycrystalline zirconia (100 vol% reinforcing phase, of 0.2–1 μm mean grain size). The imprint of microstructural features on fracture surfaces, as shown in Fig. 4.10 further indicates the fracture along internal interfaces,

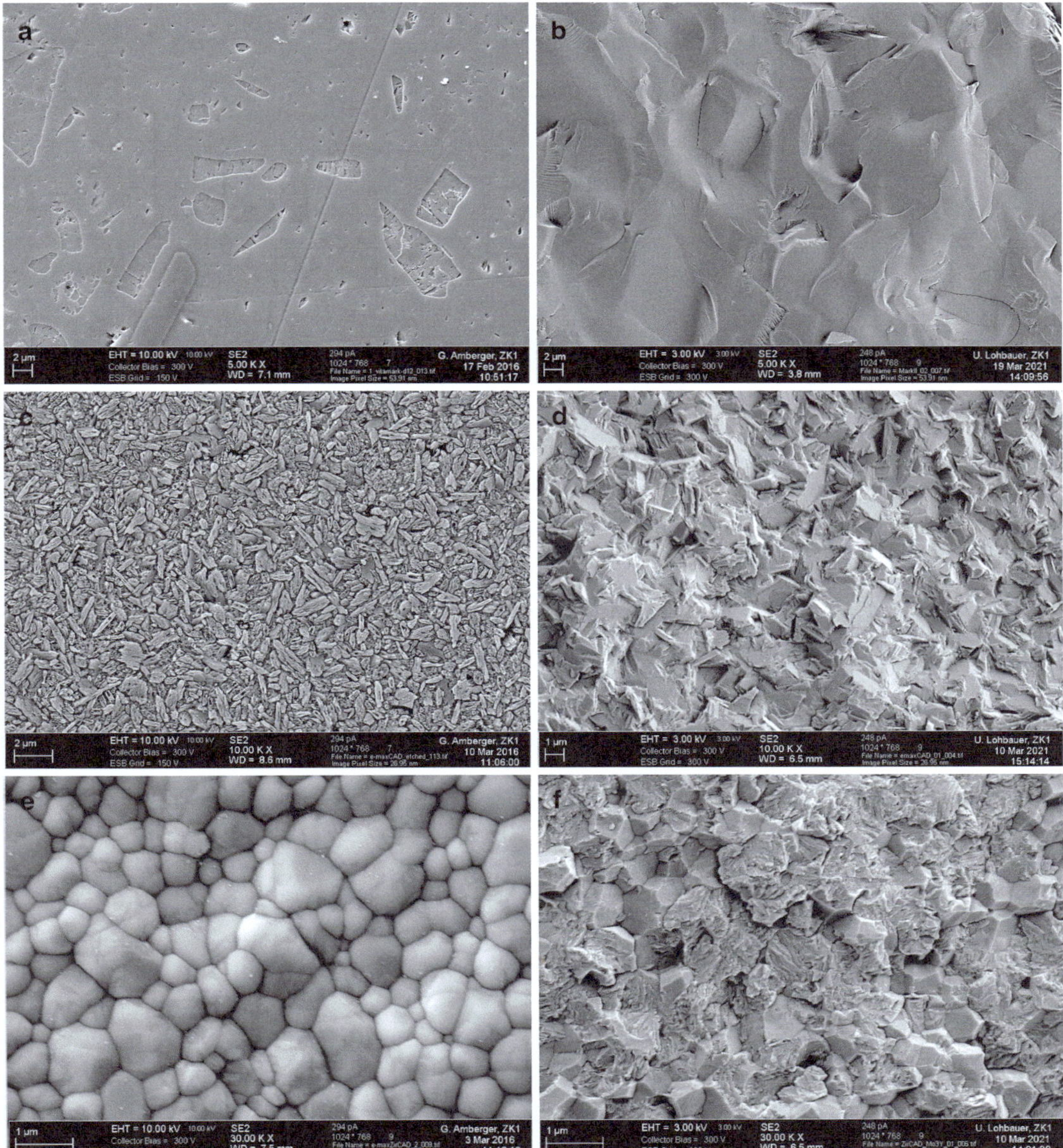

Fig. 4.10 Comparison of microstructures of three different dental ceramics with their corresponding fracture surfaces: (**a**) reinforced veneering glass (Vitablocs Mark II, Vita, albite and nepheline crystallites up to 15 μm); (**b**) the fracture surface of Vitablocs Mark II showing clear fractographic patterns (hackle lines) indicating glass fracture in the dimensional range of the reinforcing phase; (**c**) glass-ceramic (IPS e.maxCAD, Ivoclar, showing lithiumdisilicate crystallites between 1 and 2 μm); (**d**) fracture surface of IPS e.maxCAD reproducing the size and shape of the elongated lithiumdisilicate reinforcing phase; (**e**) polycrystalline 3Y-TZP zirconia (IPS e.maxZirCAD, Ivolcar, 0.2–1 μm mean grain size); and (**f**) showing the identical imprint of zirconia grains on the fracture surface, indicating an intergranular fracture mode (according to Belli et al. [11])

namely along reinforcing particles or in-between microstructural grains, indicating the preferred inter- or transgranular fracture path.

The meticulous study of fracture surfaces under high-resolution SEM imaging conditions can thus further serve as a tool for identification of the material source and fracture path.

4.2.2.2 Quantitative Fractography

The fracture toughness of a material can be measured either by crack length (stress intensity factor K_c (MPa m$^{0.5}$), by fracture energy γ_c (J/m^2), or by the strain energy release rate G_c [($G_c = 2\,\gamma_c$, according to Eq. (4.1)] [18]. Following the principles of LEFM, ceramics are most suitable materials for quantitative analysis due to the law of energy conservation during fracture. The elastically stored energy is almost completely consumed for creation of two new surfaces as a crack propagates through a material. No substantial consumption by plastic deformation or conversion into heat, acoustic or photonic energy is expected to interfere [14]. The energy release is thus a direct measure for toughness and might be correlated to the fractographic appearance and imprinted patterns [14, 19].

The relation between fracture strength of a material σ_c, its fracture toughness K_c, and the critical, fracture releasing defect size a_c are detailed described in Sect. 3.2. Based on the Griffith energy criterion, Irwin demonstrated that the material invariant constant K_c is relating the strength with the defect size as (see Sect. 3.2):

$$\sigma_c \approx a_c^{-0.5} \tag{4.3}$$

Sites of Fracture Initiation

The estimation of fracture strength via defect size measurements at a known fracture toughness becomes possible as well as vice versa calculations of fracture toughness at known fracture strength values. Equation (4.3) can either be solved by direct measurements of the fracture ori-

gin or by interpolation of a set material-inherent ratio between fracture mirror dimensions to the fracture origin, as outlined in Fig. 4.7 [20].

The fracture releasing defect is generally located in regions of maximum tensile stress, mostly found at the surface, subsurface, or edge of a specimen with extensions in two dimensions $c(x)$ and $a(y)$. Assuming a symmetric radial crack propagation, a would equal c, but in reality the crack extension is of irregular, nonsymmetric nature and the critical defect size is ultimately measured by $a_c = (ac)^{0.5}$.

Depending on the ratio between a and c, the defect size might have a circular, (semi-) elliptical, or even wider stretched shape. This in turn is influencing the geometry correction factor Y. For a circular surface defect ($c/a = 1$) the correction factor $Y = 1.29$, for a semielliptical surface defect ($c/a = 2$) the correction factor $Y = 1.24$. Such practical approximations regarding Y can be found in international standards, i.e., in EN 843-6 [1]. For a more precise calculation of the geometric factor we refer to the solutions provided by Newman and Raju [21].

An alternative approach is the measurement of fracture mirror sizes [20, 22]. Dental ceramics hardly exhibit such clear and distinct fracture initiation sites as one would find in glass. Fine, medium, or coarse-grained polycrystalline or reinforced glass ceramics do most likely not show clear and measurable indication of the fracture origin. Instead, at rather low magnifications (supported by lateral illumination), such materials exhibit a "halo" around the fracture origin. This "halo" is, however, related to a smooth to coarse transition of the fracture surface roughness indicating the mirror-mist boundary. This radius $r_{1,2,3}$ (compare Fig. 5.7) has a relation to fracture strength in terms of $\sigma_c = A/r^{0.5}$ [1, 22]. The constant A is called the mirror constant expressed in same units as the fracture toughness (MPa m$^{0.5}$). The mirror radius r thereby has a material-dependent ratio to the actual defect size

a_c between 1:6 and 1:10 [1], following $r/a_c = (A/K_{Ic})^2$ [23].

The concept of quantitative fractography has been successfully applied to dental ceramics. Della Bona et al. measured four-point fracture strength of two lithiumdisilicate materials, with variations in crystallite sizes [24]. The resulting fracture toughness was calculated based on geometric correction factors for respective surface and edge defects and according to the above Irwin criterion for fracture as shown in Eq. (4.3). The authors measured a fracture toughness of $K_{Ic} = 3.1 \pm 0.4$ MPa m$^{0.5}$ (for Li$_2$Si$_2$O$_5$ crystallite sizes between 0.5 and 2 μm) and $K_{Ic} = 3.4 \pm 0.6$ MPa m$^{0.5}$ (for Li$_2$Si$_2$O$_5$ crystallite sizes between 0.5 and 4 μm). This outcome, however, appears quite overestimated when compared to standardized fracture toughness evaluation techniques. Recent findings for the lithiumdisilicate materials IPS e.maxCAD ($K_{Ic} = 2.04$ MPa m$^{0.5}$ for Li$_2$Si$_2$O$_5$ crystallite sizes <1 μm) and IPS e.maxPress ($K_{Ic} = 2.13$ MPa m$^{0.5}$ for Li$_2$Si$_2$O$_5$ crystallite sizes between 0.2 and 4 μm) (see Table 2.2) do not confirm the above results from quantitative fractography. It seems that critical crack size radii are oversized when taken from fractographic images.

The quantitative assessment of structural defects on fracture surfaces, however, has some further limitations. Residual stress (e.g., arising at interfaces or due to cooling gradients), slow crack growth effects in humid or corrosive environments, prominent R-curve behavior, or external overlaying shear stresses are known to influence and distort the artifact dimensions [23]. In case of a nonsymmetric crack extension, it is recommended to repetitively measure the mirror-mist radius $r_{1,2,3}$ and work with the longest radius [20].

Fractal Geometry

Another approach to quantitative fractography is the use of fractal geometry of a fracture surface [25–27]. This mathematical approach to surface topography was first described by Mandelbrot [28]. Fractal objects are characterized by their fractal dimensions D. A smooth surface has a fractal dimension of $D = 2.0$. With increasing roughness or irregularity D proportionally increases to $D = 3.0$. The fractal increment $D*$ (between 0 and 1) has a theoretical correlation with the fracture toughness ($K_{Ic} \approx D^{*0.5}$) and with the mirror-mist size ratio ($D* \approx a_c/r$), respectively [27].

Hill et al. or Drummond have shown regression models for various dental ceramics with strong correlations between $D*$ and the fracture toughness K_{Ic} [25, 29]. More recently, Bulpakdi et al. or Griggs have successfully applied those principles to experimental as well as to clinically failed specimens [19, 30]. Over time, based on the protocol established by Hill et al. [25], they substantially improved the methodology as new surface inspection methods, such as atomic force microscopy (AFM) and refined software algorithms are available nowadays, making this technique a powerful tool and valuable supplement to quantitative fractography. Moreover, correlative microscopy [31] has been successfully applied to quantitative fractography.

4.2.3 Fractography of Clinical Specimens

A robust process chain toward restoration success and longevity is one ultimate goal in clinical dentistry. The highest level of evidence is gained by long-term, prospective, clinical trials, conducted in a carefully instructed and experienced team of practitioners. A helpful guidance toward proper fractographic examination of clinically retrieved specimens is described in a recent contribution [8]. Today, such clinical trials are available for most material types. However, on a less evident but broader database, systematic reviews summarize individual outcomes and manifest overall annual failure rates and respective reasons for failure. A recent prospective, multicenter, practice-based cohort study reported on clinical success of 1254 all-ceramic single crowns [32]. The authors reported an annual success rate of 92.6% and annual survival rate of 95.1% after 7.2 years in service. The main reason for failure was assigned to tooth extraction followed by ceramic fracture and defective margins. The majority of restorations were located in the premolar and molar regions finished with either a shoulder or a chamfer preparation. Interestingly, silica-based ceramics performed superior over polycrystalline ceramics and resin-based indirect composites. The overall failure rates out of such a practice-based study were naturally greater compared to prospective trials in a clinical trained environment. Earlier systematic reviews on all-ceramic single crowns as well as on all-ceramic multiple fixed partial dentures (FPDs) showed similar outcomes in terms of failure reasons [33, 34]. The annual failure rate based on 2689 Leucite/Lithiumdisilicate reinforced glass-ceramic crowns were 0.69% and that of 1049 zirconia-veneered crowns was 1.84%. The annual failure rates based on 2906 zirconia-veneered FPDs was 1.48%. Both reports in common was the significant contribution of framework, veneer or ceramic fractures to the overall failure rate, with a prominent incidence of veneer chipping for zirconia-veneered FPDs. However, the source of information regarding those clinical fractures is quite sparse. Almost no information on in situ lifetime, location of a defect, occlusal contact information, surface quality, etc., seem available. Clinical studies do rarely report on history, processing, and other related circumstances leading to individual ceramic fractures. One of our earlier works studied on correlation between clinical longevity and its predictability via parametric material properties [35]. Such attempts provide valuable insights and help bridge this gap to identify actual failure reasons and in turn help improve clinical protocols.

4.2.3.1 Fracture Types and Examples

A variety of rather case types than systematic studies have been published in order to introduce, explain, and use fractography for identification of fracture origins and explaining the underlying mechanisms. Figure 4.11 shows a random selection of clinical fractures and their counterparts in the SEM.

As restoration shape and designs are individual for each cavity preparation, the final fracture event is even more complex. Figure 4.11 shows a selection of individual reasons for clinical fractures. This list could easily be extended with numerous designs and material combinations. All in common, however, are design issues, processing deficiencies, or lack of adhesive support. In only a few cases the material itself becomes responsible for the failure, mostly we are seeing a combination of fracture reasons. Other reasons are found in clinical preparation and intraoral adjustments using rotational diamond finishing procedures. Figure 4.12a tells a story of an initially, safely designed partial inlay restoration on tooth #46. This three face mesial-occlusal-distal (MOD) inlay fractured at the bulk isthmus after 24 months in service. Due to an insufficient clinical fit, the occlusal face needed to be adjusted, hence underrunning the minimum vertical heights of 1.5 mm and in turn creating thin tapered flanges at the margins to the remaining tooth. Figure 4.12b shows an example of coarse intraoral adjustment on the occlusal face of tooth #37. The remaining defects caused by coarse rotational diamond finishing are still observable of the fracture origin site and have not been removed by successive finishing and polishing steps.

Fig. 4.11 Random examples (left column: ex situ clinical photograph; right column: corresponding SEM montage) of clinically failed restorations showing the complex nature of individual designs and defects; (**a**) and (**b**): marginal defect on a zirconia-veneered single crown on tooth # 27. The fracture occurred after 24 months in service emanating from the zirconia framework, followed by delamination of the veneer layer; (**c**) and (**d**): framework fracture of a zirconia-veneered single crown on tooth # 37. The fracture occurred after 24 months in service emanating from the zirconia framework, as indicated by the wake hackle lines in the SEM inlet; (**e**) and (**f**): marginal chippings on lithiumdisilicate crown on tooth #14 after 4 weeks in service. A combination of severe marginal machining defects and insufficient marginal fit is indicated; (**g**) and (**h**): bulk fracture of a zirconia-veneered single crown on tooth # 26 after 42 months in service. The mesial part was fractured and retrieved as a consequence of insufficient adhesive support and too thin and non-anatoform framework support; (**i**) and (**j**): marginal chipping in a glazed zirconia crown on the palatal face of tooth #17 after 36 months in service. A combination of machining defects and a thin tapered margin accounted for the fracture

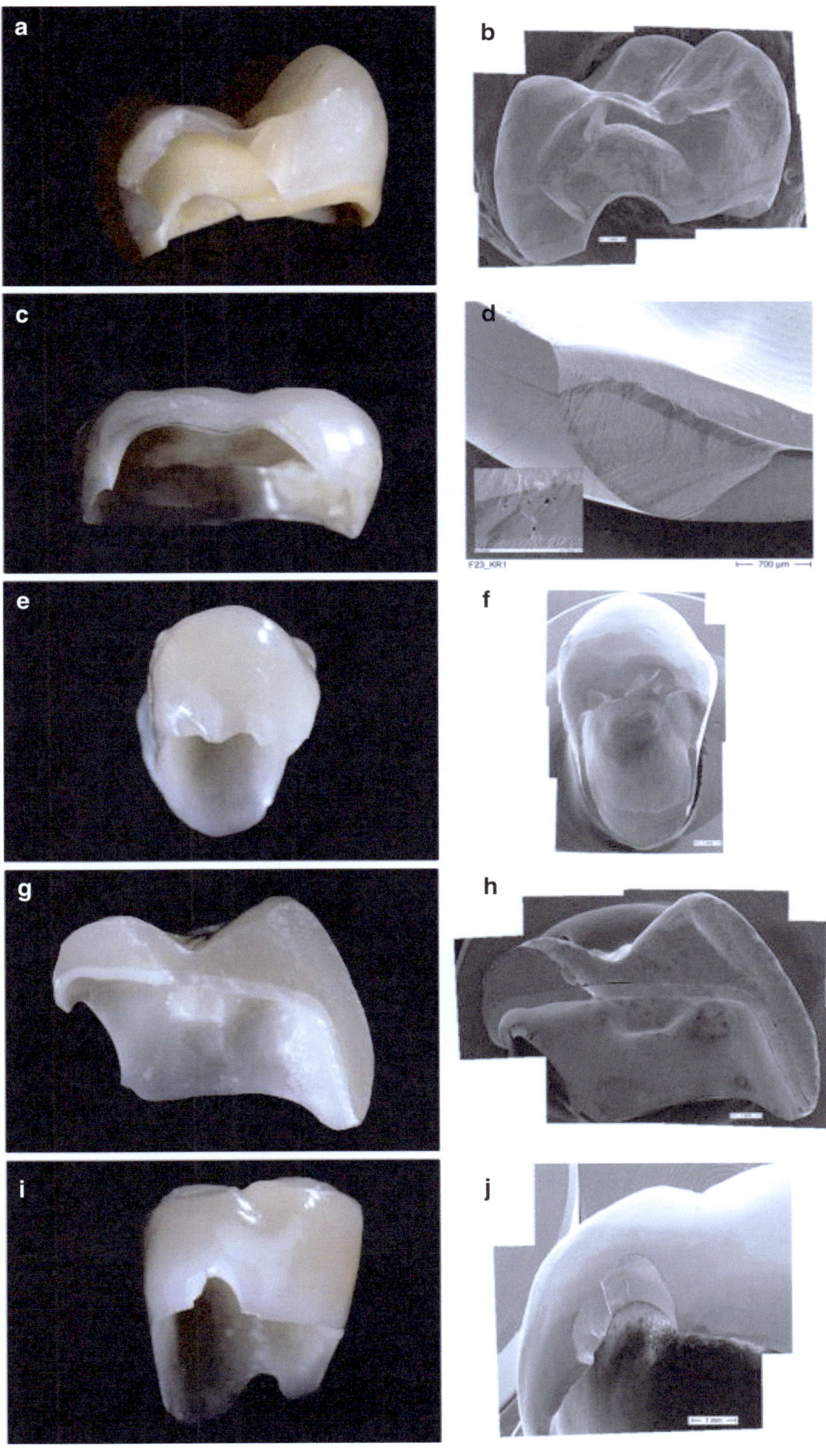

One of the first studies on clinically failed restorations was published by Kelly et al. [36]. They found either early or late fracture of ceramic crown restorations with origins emanating from the internal surface, indicating this as the highest tensile stressed or most defective region. The authors already applied quantitative fractography for estimations of stress-to-failure. Later on, Kelly et al. further investigated on failure modes comparing experimental with clinical findings [37]. Although Hertzian cone cracks were visible on the occlusal side, fractography clearly assigned connector fractures, up to 78% originating from the core-veneer interface in all-ceramic FPDs, to be the responsible failure mode in both settings. They reinforced their studies with lab strength data and numerically modelled the loading situation in order to derive suitable preparation guidance for practitioners. This example pointed out that the experimental simulation needs to meet the criteria for clinical failure. Oilo et al. later on fractographically analyzed 27 clinically fractured all-ceramic crowns and found fracture origins at the cervical margins in "the approximal area close to the most coronally placed curvature of the margin" [38]. Based on clinical fractography, one central conclusion was that fracture modes from established experimental tests were not suitably imitating the clinical situation. They developed a clinically relevant, experimental approach simulating this specific type of failure [39].

Other case studies utilizing clinical fractography as a forensic tool have pointed out various failure modes indicating the individual nature of the fracture event. A series of studies on veneered-zirconia FPDs have highlighted design issues caused by a dental technician [40], thermal incompatibilities between core and veneer materials [41], grinding damage arising from the CAD/CAM procedures [42], or even severe damage caused by patient factors such as wear and fatigue degradation of the occlusal surface [43]. The latter study gave rise to the hypothesis that veneer chipping on zirconia frameworks is not an interfacial problem but clearly located within the veneer layer and thus pointing out a prominent stress gradient perpendicular to the core-veneer interface [43]. Such examples, that surely cannot be identified from clinical inspections, clearly excavate the need for a meticulous, fractographic analysis. There is a variety of thoroughly examined cases pointing toward possible design inadequacies in either partial, single-to-multi-unit, or even implant supported restorations [44–46]. The clinical approach in common is the difficulty to identify classical fracture patterns on a broken surface. While compression curls are still clearly visible, the fracture origin in most cases is a region of damage accumulation rather than a clear mark indicating mirror, mist, and hackle regions [43]. This challenge is increasing "with the crystalline content of a material, grain size and shape, amount of transgranular and intragranular fracture, and relative size of the fractographic features" [45].

While some fractographic reports content themselves in a description of the fracture event, the actual chance of such an analysis is the analytical power to further conclude on underlying mechanisms and ultimately offer options for improvement. A recent comprehensive workup of zirconia implant design failures published by Scherrer et al. is indicating the reasons for implant fracture by analyzing the stress state and identifying the critical bending and torsion moments [46]. Considering the intraoral loading conditions, this work led to clear recommendations for improvement and finally to redesigning of the implant system used. Another example was related to the introduction of resin composite-based CAD/CAM chairside materials for subtractive milling of partial to single-unit restorations. With time after market introduction, the clinical crown indication was retracted by the manufacturer, assigning this to insufficient material properties. However, some clinical evidence were available and fractographic analysis was conducted. It turned out that not just the material properties but rather the adhesive interface was found the weakest link for those clinically fractured implant supported single crowns [47]. In another case, we worked on monolithic lithium-silicate single crowns and discovered a reproducible fracturing of such crowns during cooling from the crystallization temperature. Upon sys-

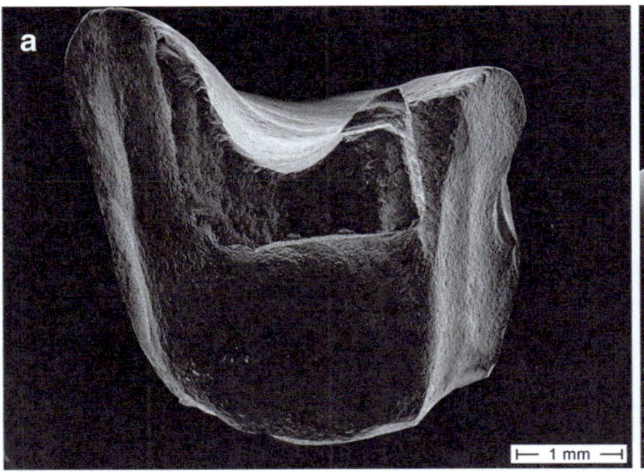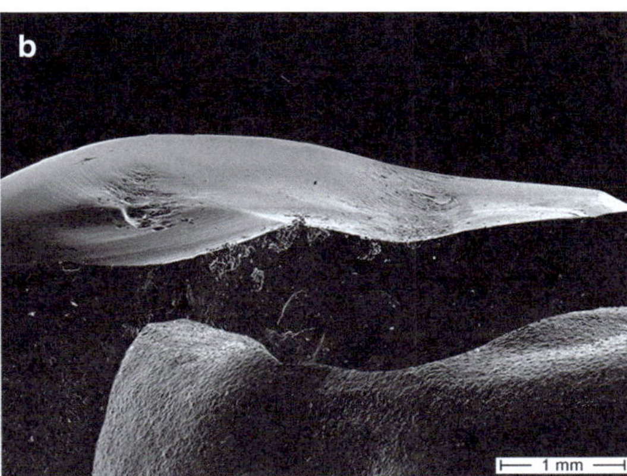

Fig. 4.12 Two examples of insufficient preparation design and intraoral adjustment procedures; (**a**) leucite reinforced MOD inlay on tooth #46 showing insufficient cross-sectional dimensions after intraoral adjustment; (**b**) fractured glass-ceramic crown on tooth #37 showing severe occlusal finishing defects on the fracture origin site

tematic analysis, we investigated and proved the hypothesis that this was due to high thermal incompatibilities between glass matrix and crystalline phases in the material and could have been prevented by reduced cooling rates [48].

However, even if those examples are helpful in identifying individual shortcomings and improving the daily practice and techniques, they still remain descriptive case reports with a limited systematic power.

Clinical fractography should not just be limited to inspection of broken surfaces, but could have a much greater power by systematic investigations. One could think of all the above-mentioned prospective clinical trials reporting on fractures as the main failure reasons but with no further effort on exploring the underlying mechanisms. Hence, a fractographer should always be connected to a clinical trial, dental practitioners should be sensitized and educated in clinical fractography, and even dental technicians should develop an understanding for material-specific preparation designs. Another systematic option could be the access and post-processing of large datasets coming out from industry-scale milling centers. Such an investigation was performed some years ago [49]. This study obtained information on approx. 35,000 restorations, produced over 3.5 years by a large CAD/CAM milling center. We retrospectively analyzed the clinical setting, material type, and other accessible aspects like cementation or surface conditioning procedures (as far as available from the dental practitioners). The company-specific warranty system for failed restorations requested a detailed description of the fracture event, the related history and time-to-failure, and most important the transmittal of broken fragments. This setting allowed us for a deep systematic analysis of 491 fractured restorations and a large-sample evaluation of high-quality data. We analyzed from partial, single-unit, and multi-unit dental restorations made from various all-ceramic materials, including leucite, lithiumdisilicate, veneered-zirconia, and even monolithic zirconia restorations. The individual material selection was however related to the respective mechanical performance and clinical indication. We analyzed clinical lifetimes and related experimental fatigue and crack growth studies and we further analyzed reasons for failure. It turned out that the majority of inspected restorations showed a combination of failure reasons, including insufficient wall thicknesses, inadequate adhesive procedures, thin tapered margins as well as coarse finishing of occlusal surfaces. Figures 4.11 and 4.12 show examples from this study pool.

4.2.3.2 Classification of Fracture Types

The previous section illustrated the individuality of each single fracture event related to the cavity situation, restoration design, processing, and clinical

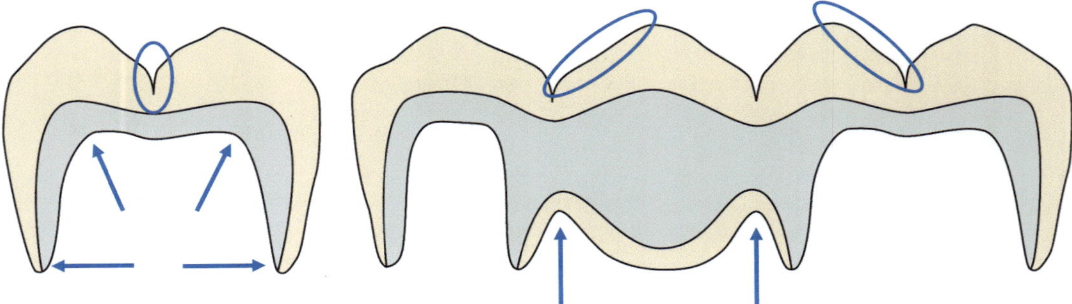

Fig. 4.13 Proposed classification of dental fracture types, modified according to Zhang and Lawn [16]

use. To further analyze and learn from such failures, it becomes inevitable to cluster and classify individual clinical fractures. Several systematic classifications of fracture modes have been proposed aiming either to distinguish the underlying mechanisms [16] or to standardize and categorize fracture events [50]. Based on their experimental expertise in contact mechanics, Zhang and Lawn derived scenarios for possible clinical crown fracture modes, including outer and inner cone cracks, chippings, and radial cracks at margins [16]. They extended their scenario to flexure cracks at bridge connectors. Figure 4.13 shows a schematic diagram indicating fracture-sensitive locations.

As presented, this is a very useful approach and the majority of the above clinical cases can be subcategorized therein.

However, such classification is based on a preceding, extensive fractographic analysis toward the respective failure modes and can hence only be used by experienced fractographers. Looking at failure reasons from a clinician's perspective, this classification is likely not applicable, as the knowledge of the underlying fracture modes is missing, based on clinical inspections. To broadly use such a classification, e.g., as assistance and guidance for prospective or other types of clinical trials, we should rather propose a system that holds for clinical prospects. Figure 4.14 presents a simple, applicable and practice-based classification system that allows clinicians to categorize their fracture types based on their inspection options using visible or microscopic tools—even a snapshot from a mobile phone might serve to identify and categorize the respective fracture type.

This proposed table is based on clinical experience in fractography. Moráguez et al. have comprehensibly visualized the relation of clinical observations to fractographic conclusions [50]. They categorized their fractures upon severity of damage into "non-critical" (repairable) and "critical" (restorable) fractures in the veneering ceramic layer or in the core structure. The three major types in Fig. 4.14 account for this general classification into veneer, core (monolithic), and core/veneer (bilayered) types. This is actually basic information that should always be provided along with any clinical reports on fractures. However, information regarding the fracture event can easily be extended toward the specific knowledge of location. The anterior or posterior region (tooth number), the individual cusp (mesial, distal), fissure, occlusal, or margin regions can further be indicated. As we are already in the middle of forensic analysis, additional information can be gathered by the support (tooth or implant) and neighboring (adjacent or opposing restorations) materials.

4.2.3.3 The Dental Replica Technique

The dental replica technique has its origins back in the eighteenth century, driven by the demand for exact replication of dental structures for restoration purposes. Today's procedure of receiving an identical twin from an inaccessible, in situ dental topography is a two-step, high precision sequence consisting of intraoral impression taking and replication via pouring the impression with a resin. The general requirement for replica materials is to ensure high precision quality with reliable, dimensional control. However, beyond

Classification	Fracture mode	Location	Specific criteria
Type I	Veneer chipping	• Incisal edge • Cusp • Fissure • Margin • contact point	• Repairable vs. restorable: cracks, chips, core exposure
Type IIa	Bulk fracture (monolithic)	• Incisor (horizontal, vertical) • Cusp, fissure (directions: mesial-distal; oral-buccal), • Margin • Bridge connector	• Adhesion vs. Cementation • Tooth vs. implant support;
Type IIb	Bulk fracture (core-veneered)		
Type III	Implant fracture	• Screw • Abutment • Implant	• Material combinations

Fig. 4.14 Proposed classification of clinical fracture types

Fig. 4.15 Consecutive dental replication protocol

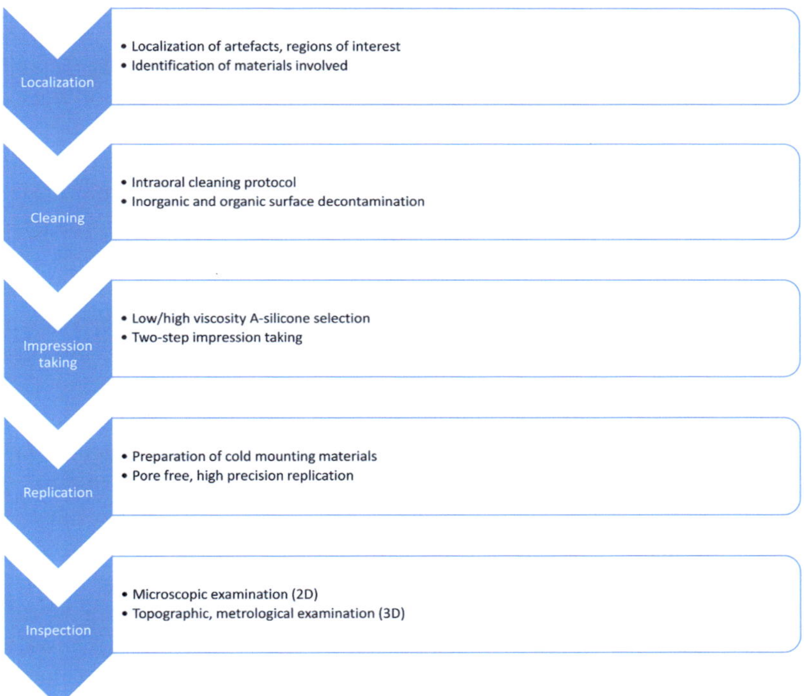

practical dental aspects, this technique offers a wide spectrum of applicability in engineering metrology and fractography. As with today's high precision and hydrophilic silicone-based impression materials, the meticulous inspection and analysis of fine microstructural features become possible. Scherrer et al. first introduced this technique for high-definition replication of fractured surfaces highlighting its use in dental fractography [51].

The common dental procedure follows a consecutive protocol as outlined in Fig. 4.15.

All steps are essential and of key relevance for a high-quality replication. For our purposes of inspection of fractured microstructures, however, some steps deserve much more attention as compared to the mandatory practical dental demands for dimensional accuracy.

The initial step for conceiving the target surface is the collection of all relevant data on processing, materials, lifetime, and the actual fracture event. Depending on the time in the mouth and exposal of the fine microstructural details to the oral environment make clear that the in situ cleaning procedure deserves special attention. Figure 4.16 lists a broad variety of cleaning agents, available to the dental practitioner. A practical recommendation is certainly the use of polymeric sponges or microbrushes for solvent application instead of pilling cotton wools (see Fig. 4.17).

In a further workflow, it becomes essential to select a hydrophilic impression material that allows perfect contact to the dry, polar region of interest. A polyaddition cross-linking A-silicone impression material is recommended over condensation-curing C-silicone materials. Figure 4.18 shows examples of suitable materials and techniques including the fine application tips of the light-body material. The two-step impression-taking technique is already implemented in dentistry and should be followed to apply a maximum hydraulic pressure to the interface between the fractured restoration surface and the light-body impression material. Figures 4.19 and 4.20 show consecutive steps of this procedure either for experimental lab specimens or for intraoral, clinical cases. A visual inspection of the impression quality is recommended to avoids any pore inclusions on the replication surface.

The next sequence in replication is the pouring of the replica material into the impression mold. The impression should be polymerized and in case of an intraoral impression taking carefully cleaned and dried. Suitable replica materials are high-definition, homogeneously mixed replica materials on the basis of polyurethane (we are using Alpha Die MF; Schütz Dental, Germany) or epoxy (Epofix, Struers) resins. The widely used material Technovit (Struers) has no high-definition potential. The use of polyether (e.g., Impregum and 3M) impression in combination with polyurethane replica materials is contraindicated as a

chemical reaction is triggered. Figure 4.21 shows the polyurethane replica material and several replication aids, useful in order to provide a pore-free contact and a perfect seal. Figure 4.22 shows the final result of the replication technique for either the clinical or the experimental technique.

The replication technique is able to provide a precise imprint of a fractured surface that might not be available for further inspection. As experimental specimens are in most cases directly available for analysis, this technique is clearly addressing the clinical, intraoral use. While retrieved broken fragments are still directly visible, chippings, wear facets, fractured restorations, and other artifacts can also be microscopically approached using the replication technique.

The final precision of the replica material is certainly the decisive factor for fractographic postprocessing. Figure 4.23 compares the fracture surface of the original, retrieved ceramic fragment with the replicated surface as to the case in Fig. 4.17a Some rounded dots are still visible on the replica (Fig. 4.23b, arrows), having its source in pore inclusions during the impression taking.

As such magnifications are certainly not sufficiently expressive and convincing for a sound fractographic inspection, Fig. 4.24 shows the fracture releasing artifact from Fig. 4.23 at a higher magnification. The replication quality allows for detailed fractographic analysis even of fine surface patterns.

A similar result can be achieved from experimental glass specimens. Figure 4.25 shows a high precision replication of a defect on a glass rod, taken from the replica in Fig. 4.22b.

Figures 4.23, 4.24, and 4.25 clearly show the potential of the dental replica technique, a powerful tool for in situ fractography of broken components that are difficult to access. In often cases there is simply one attempt possible for clinically taking an impression and the success can only be validated after final microscopic inspection. Hence, the described protocol highlights the importance for accuracy, experience, and individual training, that is mandatory for satisfying and reliable image quality.

target removal	solvent	nature	application	cave
Organic remnant removal (Biofilm, blood, saliva, collagen, smear layer)	Sodiumhypochlorit (NaClO)	Desinfection, denaturation	3%, pH=11.5, using a microbrush	Dentin/collagen denaturation
	Hydrogen peroxide (H_2O_2)	Desinfection, denaturation	3%, strong oxidizer (catalase, foaming)	Dentin/collagen denaturation, interference with subsequent intraoral adhesive repair
	Ethylenediaminetetraacetic acid (EDTA, $C_{10}H_{16}N_2O_8$)	Reduced desinfection activity, denaturation	15%, slow solvent	Dentin/collagen denaturation
Inorganic remnant removal (calcinated tissue, plaque, debris)	Phosphoric acid (H_3PO_4)	Strong acid	30-37%	Dentin & enamal etching, etching of feldspathic ceramics, no use on zirconia surfaces (interference with phosphoric primers)
	Sulfaminic acid (H_2NSO_3H)	Mild acid, decalcification	10-15%	
	Citric acid ($C_6H_8O_7$)	Mild acid	5-50%, comm. 20%	Fast and effective solvent
	Hydrofluoric acid (HF)	Strong acid	0.5-5% No buffered application	NO intraoral use! Only for zirconia surfaces! Silica based ceramic etching
Bacteria, pathogens	Chloramin-T	Desinfection	0.5%, storage desinfection for extracted teeth	No use for cleaning purposes
	Chlorhexidine	Desinfection	0.1-2%	No use for cleaning purposes, never in combination with NaOCL (chloraniline!)
	Tubulicid (blue label, Dental therapeutics))	Amphotenside, pH=7.3, Desinfection	Cavity cleaning	No use for cleaning purposes
Cement remnant removal	Ivoclean (Ivoclar; NaOH)	Universal cleaning, pH=13-13.5	General restoration cleaning, extraoral use	Acid etching of feldspathic ceramics
	Temp:ex (Renfert, KOH)	Alkaline and universal cleaning, pH=13-14	Cement removal	Acid etching of feldspathic ceramics
General purpose (hydrophilic & hydrophobic remnants)	Ethanol (C_2H_6O)	Amphiphilic solvent, dipole molecule	99,5%	Always recommended step
	Water	Neutral solvent	Water spray	Distilled or deionized water
	Air	Drying agent	Compressed air	Oil free air
Gold sputter coating romoval	Potassium triiodide (Lugol's iodine (I_2/KI); TechniEtch ACl2 (microchemicals.com))		5%	Extraoral use only
Silicone oil removal	Petroleum ether			Removal of remnants from silicone impressions for further adhesive procedure, extraoral use!

Fig. 4.16 Cleaning agents used in the dental practice for effective removal of specific remnants

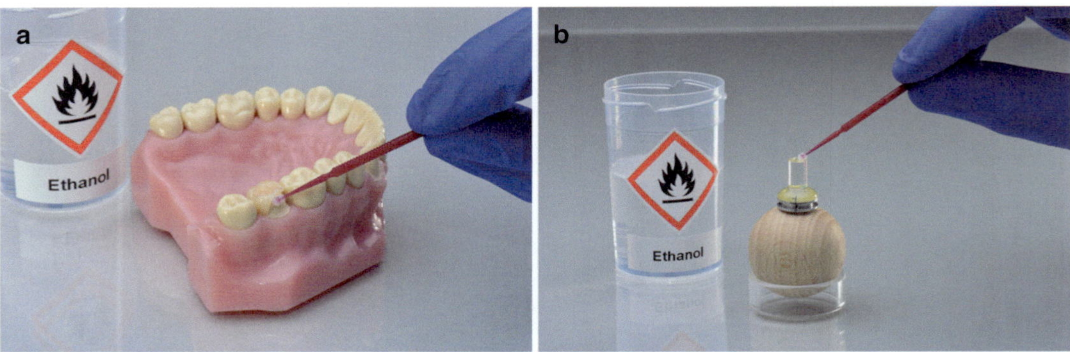

Fig. 4.17 The dental cleaning procedure using a cleaning agent (here: ethanol) and a microbrush; (**a**) application on clinical cases, (**b**) application on lab specimens

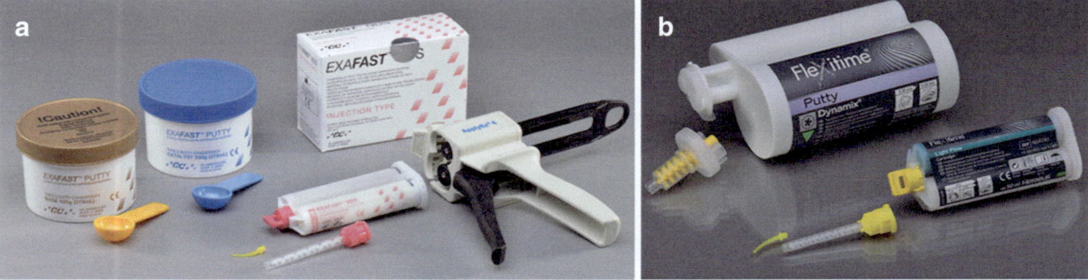

Fig. 4.18 Examples of impression material selection; (**a**) putty version; (**b**) application of the heavy-body impression material in automix cartridges. The 2K light-body materials are commonly delivered in automix syringes, equipped with an extruder and a fine application tip

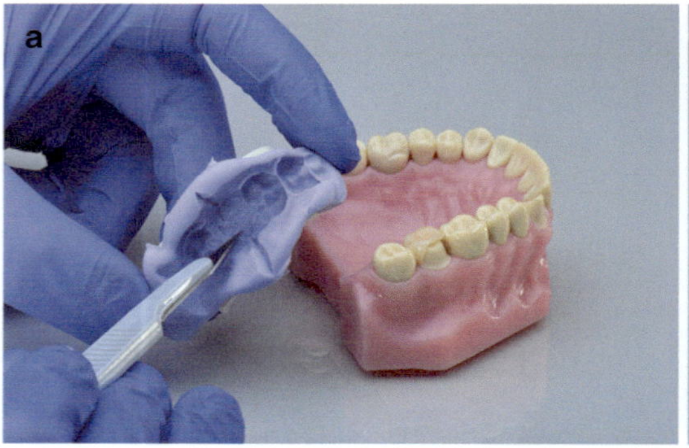
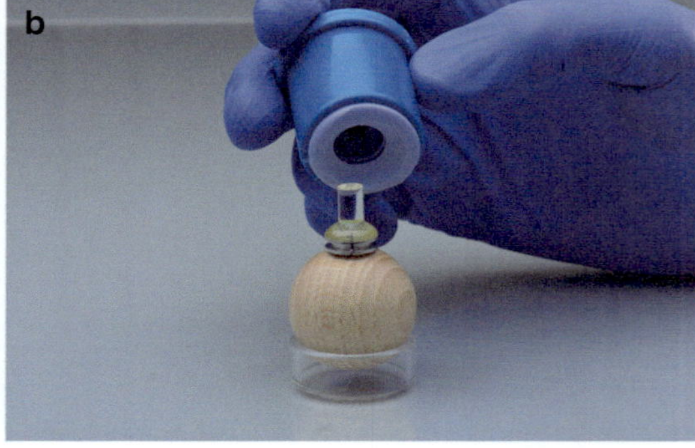

Fig. 4.19 First step of impression taking using a heavy-body A-silicone in order to provide dimensional stability to the impression; (**a**) clinical procedure using minitrays and showing the trimming step using a sharp scalpel; (**b**) mold support for the heavy-body impression

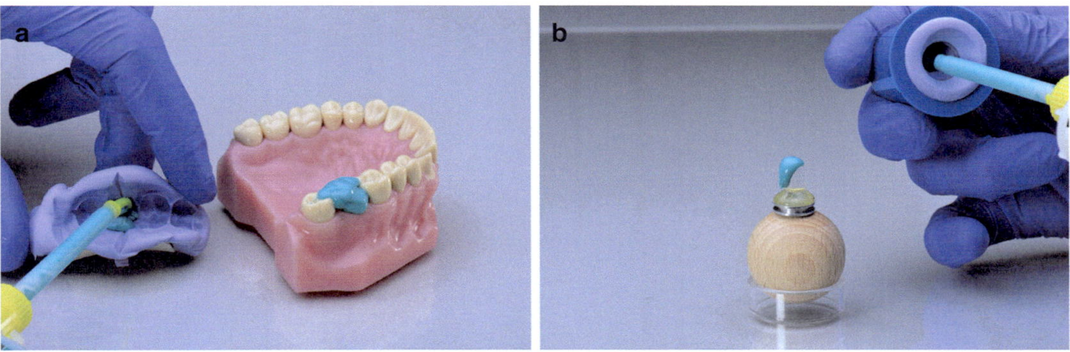

Fig. 4.20 Application of the high-precision light-body impression material on both surfaces; (**a**) clinical procedure, (**b**) experimental procedure

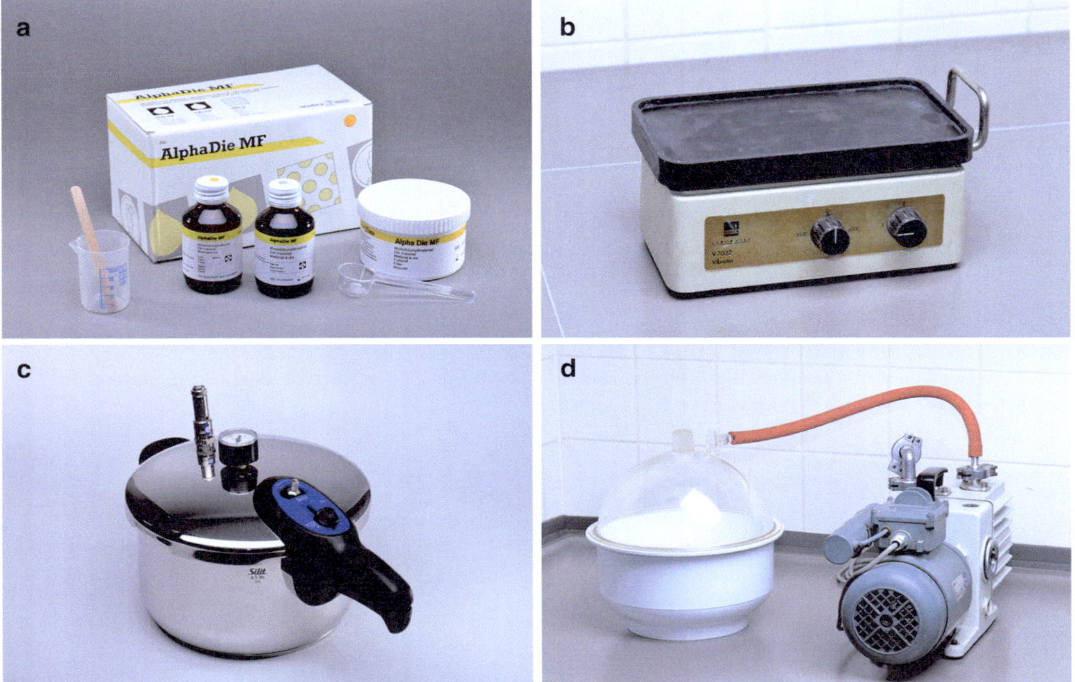

Fig. 4.21 Example of a polyurethane replica material (**a**) used by dental technicians and important processing aids, such as a vibration device (**b**), pressure vessel (**c**), or a vacuum exsiccator (**d**) in order to minimize any residual porosity on the replicated surface

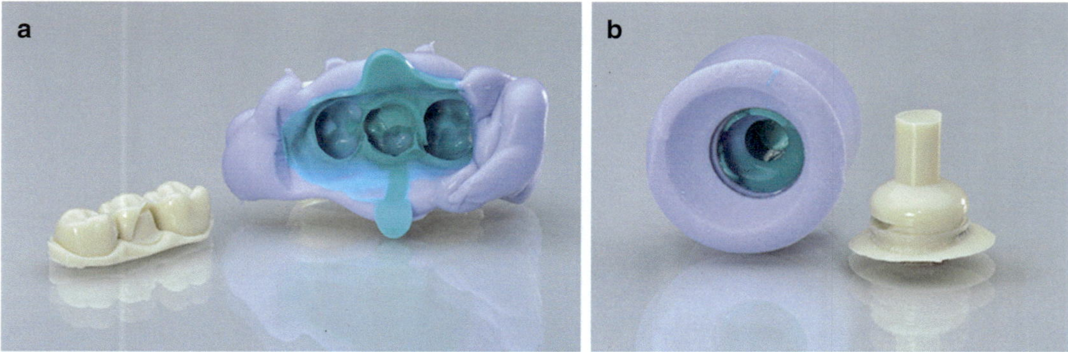

Fig. 4.22 Final replication of the target surface using a polyurethane, cold-mounting replica material; (**a**) intraoral procedure, (**b**) experimental procedure

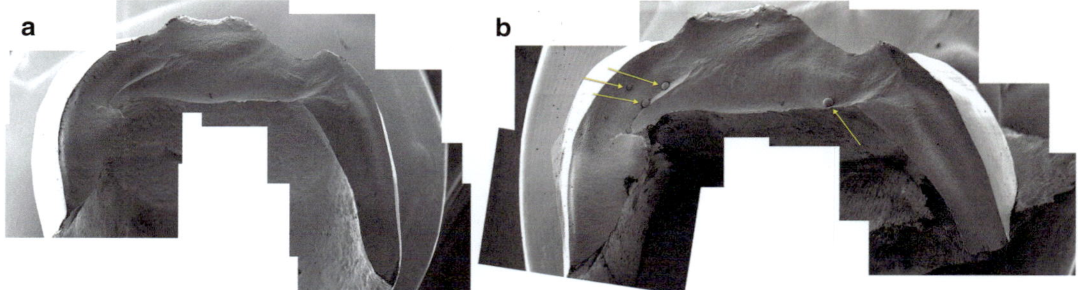

Fig. 4.23 Reconstructed set of SEM images of the fracture surface of a clinically fractured dental crown from (**a**) original, retrieved ceramic fragment, and (**b**) replicated surface using the described technique. Processing pores are observable on the replicated surface (arrows)

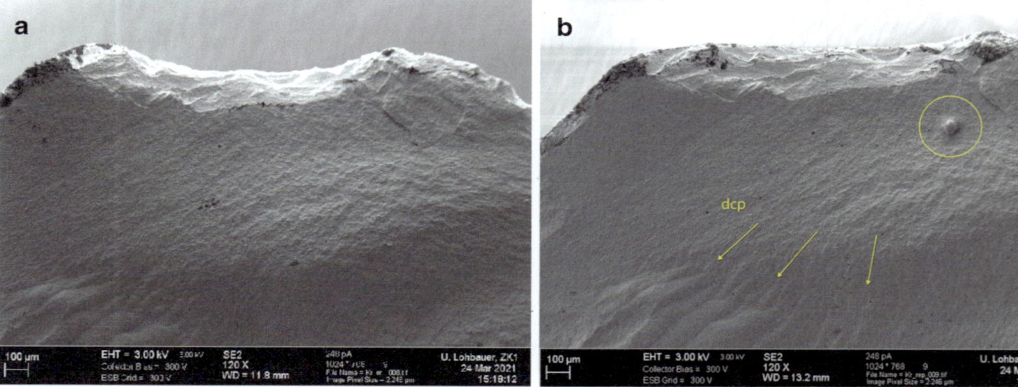

Fig. 4.24 SEM images from fracture releasing region on the occlusal side of the dental crown. Fine hackle marks are visible on both the original surface (**a**) and the replicated surface (**b**, arrows). A processing pore is observable on the replicated surface (circle)

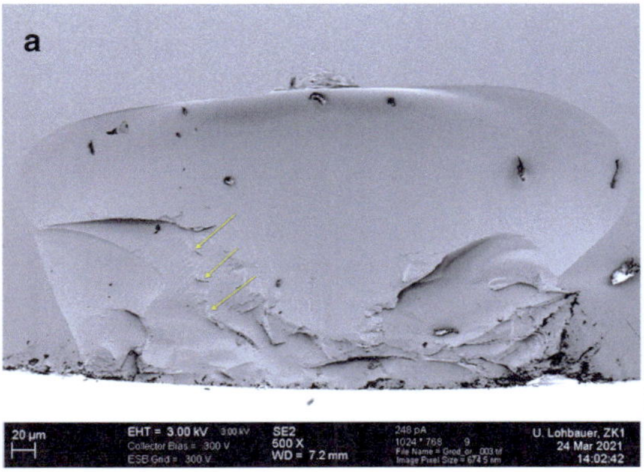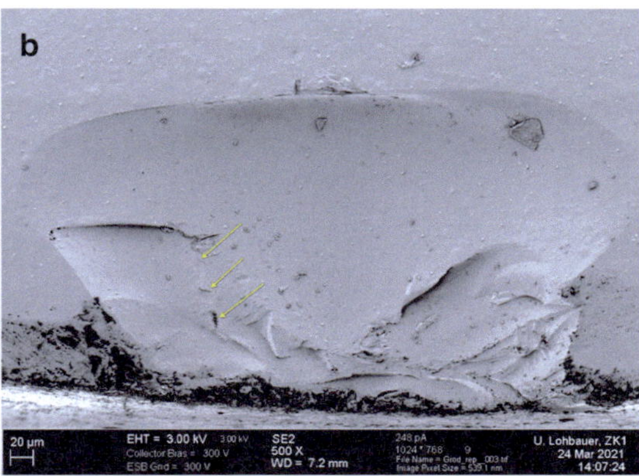

Fig. 4.25 SEM image of a fracture pattern identified at a glass rod at 500x magnification. Still, some locally defined replication artifacts are observable (**b**) compared to the original surface (**a**). Fine hackle lines however are observable on both surfaces (arrows)

References

1. EN 843-6. Advanced technical ceramics—mechanical properties of monolithic ceramics at room temperature—part 6: guidance for fractographic investigation. Brussels: European committee for standardization (CEN); 2009.
2. ASTM C1322-15. Standard practice for fractography and characterization of fracture origins in advanced ceramics. West Conshohocken: ASTM International; 2015.
3. Quinn GD. On terminal crack velocities in glasses. Int J Appl Glas Sci. 2019;10(1):7–16.
4. Griffith AA. The phenomena of rupture and flow in solids. Philos Trans R Soc Lond A. 1921;221:163–98.
5. Quinn GD. NIST recommended practice guide: Fractography of ceramics and glasses. 3rd ed. Gaithersburg, MD: National Institute of Standards and Technology; 2020.
6. EN 843-1. Advanced technical ceramics—mechanical properties of monolithic ceramics at room temperature—part 1: determination of flexural strength. Brussels: European committee for standardization (CEN); 2008.
7. Quinn JB, Quinn GD. A practical and systematic review of Weibull statistics for reporting strengths of dental materials. Dent Mater. 2010;26(2):135–47.
8. Scherrer SS, Lohbauer U, Della Bona A, Vichi A, Tholey MJ, Kelly JR, et al. ADM guidance-ceramics: guidance to the use of fractography in failure analysis of brittle materials. Dent Mater. 2017;33(6):599–620.
9. Wendler M, Belli R, Petschelt A, Mevec D, Harrer W, Lube T, et al. Chairside CAD/CAM materials. Part 2: flexural strength testing. Dent Mater. 2017;33(1):99–109.
10. Harrer W, Morrell R, Danzer R. Fractography of biaxial tested Si3N4-specimens. J Eur Ceram Soc. 2014;34(14):3283–9.
11. Belli R, Wendler M, de Ligny D, Cicconi MR, Petschelt A, Peterlik H, et al. Chairside CAD/CAM materials. Part 1: measurement of elastic constants and microstructural characterization. Dent Mater. 2017;33(1):84–98.
12. Belli R, Wendler M, Petschelt A, Lube T, Lohbauer U. Fracture toughness testing of biomedical ceramic-based materials using beams, plates and discs. J Eur Ceram Soc. 2018;38(16):5533–44.
13. Morrell R. Measurement good practice guide no. 15—Fractography of brittle materials. Teddington: National Physical Laboratory; 1999.
14. Bradt RC. The fractography and crack patterns of broken glass. J Fail Anal Prev. 2011;11(2):79–96.
15. Wiederhorn SM. Influence of water vapor on crack propagation in soda-lime glass. J Am Ceram Soc. 1967;50(8):407–14.
16. Zhang Y, Sailer I, Lawn BR. Fatigue of dental ceramics. J Dent. 2013;41(12):1135–47.
17. Wendler M, Belli R, Valladares D, Petschelt A, Lohbauer U. Chairside CAD/CAM materials. Part 3: cyclic fatigue parameters and lifetime predictions. Dent Mater. 2018;34(6):910–21.
18. Mecholsky JJ Jr. Fracture mechanics principles. Dent Mater. 1995;11(2):111–2.
19. Griggs JA. Using fractal geometry to examine failed implants and prostheses. Dent Mater. 2018;34(12):1748–55.
20. Mecholsky JJ Jr. Fractography: determining the sites of fracture initiation. Dent Mater. 1995;11(2):113–6.
21. Newman JC, Raju IS. An empirical stress-intensity factor equation for the surface crack. Eng Fract Mech. 1981;15(1):185–92.
22. Kirchner HP, Kirchner JW. Fracture mechanics of fracture mirrors. J Am Ceram Soc. 1979;62(3–4):198–202.

23. Marshall DB, Lawn BR, Mecholsky JJ. Effect of residual contact stresses on mirror/flaw-size relations. J Am Ceram Soc. 1980;63(5–6):358–60.
24. Della Bona A, Mecholsky JJ Jr, Anusavice KJ. Fracture behavior of lithia disilicate- and leucite-based ceramics. Dent Mater. 2004;20(10):956–62.
25. Hill TJ, Della Bona A, Mecholsky JJ Jr. Establishing a protocol for measurements of fractal dimensions in brittle materials. J Mater Sci. 2001;36(11):2651–7.
26. Mecholsky JJ, Passoja DE, Feinberg-Ringel KS. Quantitative analysis of brittle fracture surfaces using fractal geometry. J Am Ceram Soc. 1989;72(1):60–5.
27. Mecholsky JJ Jr, Freiman SW. Relationship between fractal geometry and fractography. J Am Ceram Soc. 1991;74(12):3136–8.
28. Mandelbrot BB. The fractal geometry of nature. New York: W.H. Freeman; 1982.
29. Drummond JL, Thompson M, Super BJ. Fracture surface examination of dental ceramics using fractal analysis. Dent Mater. 2005;21(6):586–9.
30. Bulpakdi P, Taskonak B, Yan J, Mecholsky JJ Jr. Failure analysis of clinically failed all-ceramic fixed partial dentures using fractal geometry. Dent Mater. 2009;25(5):634–40.
31. Hein LR, de Oliveira JA, de Campos KA. Correlative fractography: combining scanning electron microscopy and light microscopes for qualitative and quantitative analysis of fracture surfaces. Microsc Microanal. 2013;19(2):496–500.
32. Wierichs RJ, Kramer EJ, Reiss B, Schwendicke F, Krois J, Meyer-Lueckel H, et al. A prospective, multi-center, practice-based cohort study on all-ceramic crowns. Dent Mater. 2021;37(8):1273–82.
33. Pjetursson BE, Sailer I, Makarov NA, Zwahlen M, Thoma DS. All-ceramic or metal-ceramic tooth-supported fixed dental prostheses (FDPs)? A systematic review of the survival and complication rates. Part II: Multiple-unit FDPs. Dent Mater. 2015;31(6):624–39.
34. Sailer I, Makarov NA, Thoma DS, Zwahlen M, Pjetursson BE. All-ceramic or metal-ceramic tooth-supported fixed dental prostheses (FDPs)? A systematic review of the survival and complication rates. Part I: single crowns (SCs). Dent Mater. 2015;31(6):603–23.
35. Lohbauer U, Kramer N, Petschelt A, Frankenberger R. Correlation of in vitro fatigue data and in vivo clinical performance of a glassceramic material. Dent Mater. 2008;24(1):39–44.
36. Kelly JR, Giordano R, Pober R, Cima MJ. Fracture surface analysis of dental ceramics: clinically failed restorations. Int J Prosthodont. 1990;3(5):430–40.
37. Kelly JR, Tesk JA, Sorensen JA. Failure of all-ceramic fixed partial dentures in vitro and in vivo: analysis and modeling. J Dent Res. 1995;74(6):1253–8.
38. Oilo M, Gjerdet NR. Fractographic analyses of all-ceramic crowns: a study of 27 clinically fractured crowns. Dent Mater. 2013;29(6):e78–84.
39. Oilo M, Kvam K, Tibballs JE, Gjerdet NR. Clinically relevant fracture testing of all-ceramic crowns. Dent Mater. 2013;29(8):815–23.
40. Lohbauer U, Amberger G, Quinn GD, Scherrer SS. Fractographic analysis of a dental zirconia framework: a case study on design issues. J Mech Behav Biomed Mater. 2010;3(8):623–9.
41. Lohbauer U, Belli R, Arnetzl G, Scherrer SS, Quinn GD. Fracture of a veneered-ZrO2 dental prosthesis from an inner thermal crack. Case Stud Eng Fail Anal. 2014;2(2):100–6.
42. Belli R, Scherrer SS, Lohbauer U. Report on fractures of trilayered all-ceramic fixed dental prostheses. Case Stud Eng Fail Anal. 2016;7:71–9.
43. Belli R, Scherrer SS, Reich S, Petschelt A, Lohbauer U. In vivo shell-like fractures of veneered-ZrO2 fixed dental prostheses. Case Stud Eng Fail Anal. 2014;2(2):91–9.
44. Quinn GD, Hoffman K, Scherrer S, Lohbauer U, Amberger G, Karl M, et al. Fractographic analysis of broken ceramic dental restorations. Ceramic Transactions; 2012. p. 161–74.
45. Scherrer SS, Quinn JB, Quinn GD, Kelly JR. Failure analysis of ceramic clinical cases using qualitative fractography. Int J Prosthodont. 2006;19(2):185–92.
46. Scherrer SS, Mekki M, Crottaz C, Gahlert M, Romelli E, Marger L, et al. Translational research on clinically failed zirconia implants. Dent Mater. 2019;35(2):368–88.
47. Lohbauer U, Belli R, Cune MS, Schepke U. Fractography of clinically fractured, implant-supported dental computer-aided design and computer-aided manufacturing crowns. SAGE Open Med Case Rep. 2017;5:2050313X17741015.
48. Lohbauer U, Wendler M, Rapp D, Belli R. Fractographic analysis of lithium silicate crown failures during sintering. SAGE Open Med Case Rep. 2019;7:2050313X19838962.
49. Belli R, Petschelt A, Hofner B, Hajto J, Scherrer SS, Lohbauer U. Fracture rates and lifetime estimations of CAD/CAM all-ceramic restorations. J Dent Res. 2016;95(1):67–73.
50. Moraguez OD, Wiskott HW, Scherrer SS. Three- to nine-year survival estimates and fracture mechanisms of zirconia- and alumina-based restorations using standardized criteria to distinguish the severity of ceramic fractures. Clin Oral Investig. 2015;19(9):2295–307.
51. Scherrer SS, Quinn JB, Quinn GD, Wiskott HW. Fractographic ceramic failure analysis using the replica technique. Dent Mater. 2007;23(11):1397–404.

Construction and design principles for dental prostheses are a wide and extremely individual, specific field in engineering design. Each dental cavity preparation is unique in shape, extension, depth, and orientation. This chapter fills an important gap in education of dental practitioners, of which the quintessence is summarized in respective clinical preparation guidelines.

However, since material innovations are on the fast lane and new treatment strategies enter the dental world by reaching out to the practitioner, the profound knowledge in construction design and principles and the underlying mechanisms becomes as important as the understanding of load transfer through a restored tooth or prosthesis.

Not just the basic material properties, ranking one material to another, or processing guidelines for proper placement are henceforth sufficient, but more the holistic understanding of the oral situation, the occlusion in the context of neighbor and antagonist teeth, and the mutual action of load or stress and the expected reaction in form of deformation or strain of a compound comes into focus of a sound and stable restorative treatment. The knowledge of maximum applied stress and regions of stress concentration within a restorative compartment is essential for the prevention of any type of fatigue or spontaneous failure.

This chapter is combining the oral boundaries in mastication with principles in engineering design, thereby reflecting on load transfer and compliance through a loaded dentition. Basic, biomimetic, and individual concepts are explained on a variety of applied, practical examples.

5.1 Clinical Boundaries

5.1.1 Oral Physiology

Mastication is a process that is driven by the opening and closing movement of the lower jaw, the mandible. This jaw is connected to the temporal bone of the skull (cranium) through the temporomandibular joint (TMJ; also called craniomandibular joint (CMJ)). The two condyles on both sides of the TMJ thereby ensure a maximum mobility of the mandible during mastication. Together with the dentition in occlusion, the mandible outlines the articulatory system and fulfills its primary task: controlled crushing preparation of the food bolus and swallowing for further digestion.

The masticatory process, however, is an interplay of opening and closing sequences, guided by the sensitive neuromuscular activity of the mandibular jaw. The grade of freedom in jaw mobility was first described by Dr. Ulf Posselt, who already back in 1952 introduced a 3D concept of mandibular movements [1]. This concept described boarder movements in the frontal, horizontal, and sagittal planes and became the standard concept in

---

The original version of the chapter has been revised. A correction to this chapter can be found at https://doi.org/10.1007/978-3-030-94687-6_6

prosthodontics, better known as "Posselt's envelope of motion" [2]. While anatomical differences between individuals are biologically normal, the concept generally holds for principle movements and the chewing loop is well seated within this envelope. Figure 5.1 shows the boarder movements in the three planes and indicates the chewing kinematics as not just simple vertical movements.

The masticatory cycle is characterized by an opening and closing phase with the resting position one the one end and the power stroke on the other end of the cycle [3]. The shape of this extremely individual hysteresis is well seated within the envelope of motion and controlled by the masticatory and occlusal system, as well as by factors such as gender or variations in food hardness and volume [3, 4]. During chewing, the mandible returns into its preferred reference positions: the centric relation point, the maximum intercuspal position, and the postural position. The centric relation or centric occlusion is a physiologically and biologically preferred (natural) jaw position in which the occlusal contacts are in harmony and fully seated with the opposing dentition. Ideally, the centric occlusion may coincide with the maximum intercuspal position, the position with maximum contacts on the occlusal surface [5]. In case of deviations from that concept, teeth might be subjected to premature contacts before reaching the maximum intercuspation. This in turn might result in overloading, discomfort, wear, fatigue, or even fracture [5].

The mandible generally moves in rotational and transversal modes against the maxilla (upper jaw). During closing movement, the mandible deviates laterally toward the working side (the side to which the mandible is moving) while the muscles counteract on the balancing side (opposite the working side). Maximum intercuspation is not yet reached as the food bolus is still under digestion. The final power stroke continues to move the mandible toward maximum intercuspation with all occlusal contacts in position [5].

5.1.2 Occlusion and Load Transfer

The term "occlusion" is defined as the "static relationship between the incising or masticating surfaces of the maxillary or mandibular teeth or tooth analogues" [6]. The closing movement in the masticatory cycle is the relevant step for considerations toward construction and design of restoration as load is transferred between the opposing dentitions in occlusion. The neuromuscular control of chewing is responsible for the chewing sequence (closed-loop control). The kinematic process is driven by muscle contraction and load application until the final power stroke at maximum intercuspation. Sensitive mechanoreceptors, especially located in the periodontal ligament (PMRs), provide information for the central nervous system and hence account

Fig. 5.1 Posselt's envelope of motion in frontal, horizontal, and sagittal planes (*ICP* maximum intercuspation point, *RCP* centric relation point, *O* maximum opening, *Pr* maximum protrusion, *L* left laterotrusion, *R* right laterotrusion, *P* postural position)

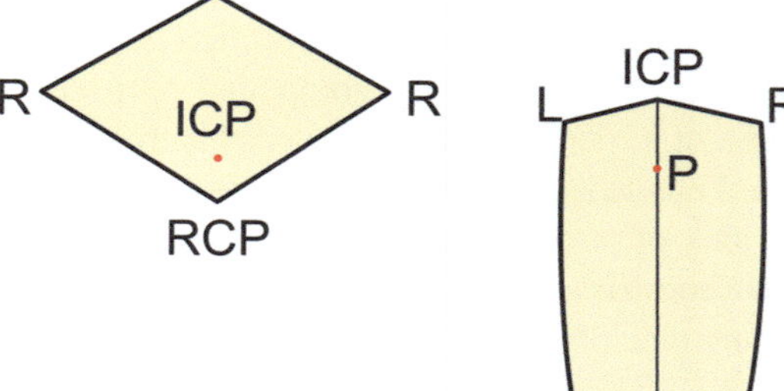

for unloading and occlusal release [7]. The jaw opening reflex, a protection against sudden contacts or overloading, is an important feature in the neuromuscular control, available, however, only for vital teeth [5]. PMRs further control a certain tactual sensibility between the opposing dentitions [8]. Particles larger than 10–15 µm can be perceived by sound teeth while this threshold value is found reduced with increasingly invasive replacements from crowns, bridges to even total prosthesis usually ranging from 20 to 100 µm [5, 9].

A central factor regarding the stress transferred to a tooth or prosthesis in occlusion is the build-up of bite forces. The dental scientific literature provides us with extensive outcomes on bite force measurements, however, associated with a high scatter of data [10]. Experimental approaches including gnathodynamometers, strain-gauges, and optical and piezoelectric sensors are described in literature as well as the virtual, numeric simulation of the masticatory system [10, 11]. A comprehensive review of the scientific literature toward assessment of physiological and pathological bite forces has been published by Röhrle et al. [10].

Posterior teeth in maximum intercuspation indicate maximum bite forces of up to 300–400 N [5, 10]. Anterior teeth are thereby subjected to lower vertical loads, as the mandible closing moment is reduced compared to the shorter posterior region. Such data, however, are highly dependent on individual factors like age, gender, habits, and occlusal situation. Extreme scatter data might hence be statistically treated or mathematically smoothened and averaged via, e.g., Fourier series [12]. Over time, the multiplicity of studies provides a reliable picture of bite forces, as summarized in the above-mentioned review [10]. During chewing or grinding, lateral shear forces overlay the vertical bite force [13]. Pathological bite forces, on the other hand, are arising from daily or overnight bruxing (parafunctional grinding of teeth), gnashing, or clenching. This field is even more complex as multifactorial reasons might contribute to this pathological habit. Among crucial factors, occlusal disharmony or the individual stress level is

named at first place. Bite forces during clenching or bruxing are far greater compared to the physiological range. It is reported that the level of vertical bite forces might increase up to 3–10 times the physiological range [5].

As simple as physics can be, the stress effects on the surface is a function of the bite force divided by the occlusal contact area, i.e., by the number of point contacts. Approximately 80% of the total bite force is distributed in the posterior region [13].

Figure 5.2 shows an example of ideal occlusal intercuspation on a first molar tooth showing seven major contact points. The contact points are located on the cusp planes. Figure 5.2 further shows that a single tooth has contact with two opposing teeth (a main and a side antagonist), sometimes termed as "tooth-to-two-tooth" contact, with additional contact points on marginal ridges.

As occlusal contacts determine the stress distribution between opposing dentitions, a harmonic occlusion is the ultimate goal in functional anatomy. Practical criteria are a maximum contact area (in order to optimize the masticatory effort), the orientation of teeth along the vertical tooth axis, the position of opposing teeth (functional cusps should occlude with the antagonist

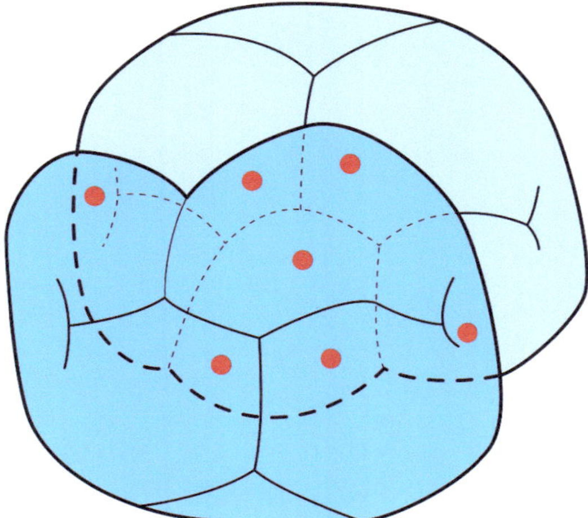

Fig. 5.2 Maximum of shared occlusal contact points of a molar tooth in harmonic occlusion, according to [9]

fossa or marginal ridge), and a simultaneous, uniform contact on all occlusal contact points [9].

The occlusal surface of a posterior tooth generally consists of cusps, fissures, and marginal ridges. Figure 5.3 shows the complex intercuspation where cusps of the one enter the fissure of the other tooth. Figure 5.3 schematically draws the occlusal intercuspation of the upper and lower first molars. The upper palatal cusp as well as the lower buccal cusp are the functional (centric) cusps, extending into the opposing fossa. The dimension of the functional cusp is commonly wider compared to the non-functional, so-called shear cusp. On each molar tooth, the anatomically relevant area of chewing is circumscribed by the cusps and the marginal ridges. Both, the palatal as well as the buccal slopes of the functional cusps are involved in occlusion. Figure 5.3 further shows the tooth axis along which forces

are transduced in harmonic occlusion. Assuming a lateral closing movement of the mandible during mastication induces a prominent overlay of shear forces in palatal direction [5, 9]. The maximum intercuspation is, however, still limited by point contacts. Fissures remain open as their function is to incise, comminute, and transport the food bolus.

Occlusion, however, is not just defined by static contact points, as outlined in Fig. 5.2, but is further guided by dynamic occlusion. Off-axis loading in terms of eccentric mandibular movement during chewing or even during severe parafunctional grinding or bruxing might happen in laterotrusional, mediotrusional, or protrusional directions, resulting in considerable shear stress against the tooth axis.

5.1.3 Compliance of Oral Structures

The masticatory load that is accumulated on the occlusal surface and transduced through the tooth, restoration, or a prosthesis, is the crucial factor regarding mechanical construction and stability. Focusing on the local neighborhood of two opposing posterior teeth, as shown in Fig. 5.3, the system offers a certain compliance against vertical or even lateral forces. This compliance is due to the viscoelastic and hydrodynamic damping properties of the periodontal ligament (PDL) in the beginning and on the elastic properties of dentin and enamel at the end of the masticatory closing cycle.

Every single tooth is flexibly mounted in its respective alveolus. A membrane of connective tissue fiber bundles thereby holds the tooth in position (syndesmosis). Those type-I-collagen fibers are also called Sharpey's fibers. Figure 5.4 schematically shows the fibrous tooth attachment to the alveolar bone.

Multiple fiber bundles have the ability to resist external forces in relation to their respective orientations. While horizontal fibers are mainly effective to resist lateral or shear forces, oblique fiber bundles are the main component to resist vertical and intrusive forces. The space between tooth and bone is measuring approxi-

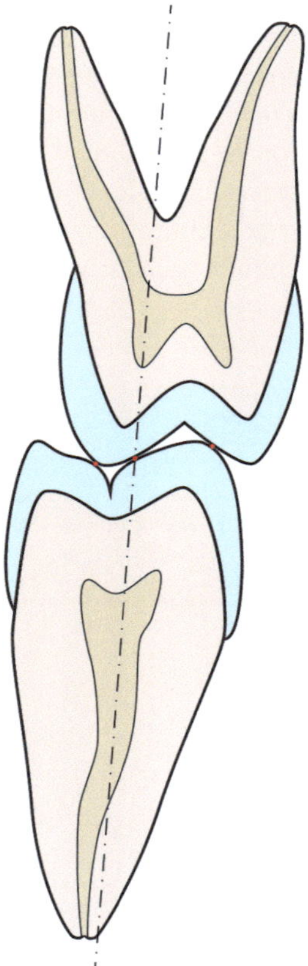

Fig. 5.3 Two opposing first molar teeth in occlusion aligned along their tooth axis, according to [9]

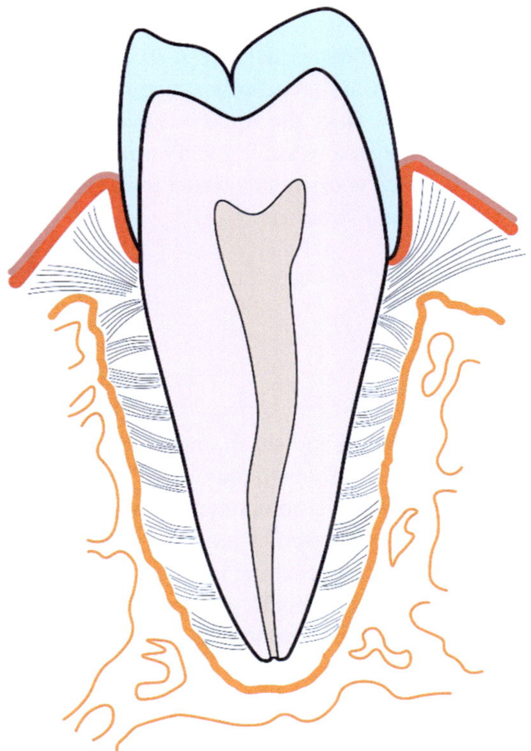

Fig. 5.4 A posterior tooth attached to the alveolar bone. Alveolar crest fibers run from the cervical root part toward the alveolar crest; horizontal fibers run from the cementum horizontal to the alveolar bone; Oblique fibers run from the cementum to the alveolar bone in an oblique direction; periapical fibers are radially extending from the apex to the alveolar bone, according to [14, 15]

mately 0.25 mm at the alveolar crest to 0.1 mm at the central section [5]. Based on this setting, a sound tooth is able to offer a compliant compressive strain against external forces in axial as well as in lateral directions. Tooth mobility studies have measured a deflection range between 50-100 μm at external loading of 2–5 N [9]. This, however, depends on the anterior or posterior location with reduced mobility in the posterior region. Due to the fact that posterior teeth offer a far (twice) larger root surface area the toughening effect is even superior compared to front teeth.

This "shock-absorbing" effect, however, is lost, when replacing a natural tooth by an implant. A finally osseointegrated implant builds a rigid, intimate contact with the surrounding bone tissue and cannot follow the neuromuscular response during mastication as relevant mechanoreceptors are removed [5, 15]. Comparing the chewing patterns on natural versus implant-supported teeth prosthesis, differences in muscle activity have been observed, in the way of lacking sensitivity on implant supports during mastication [16]. In order to compensate for this lack of sensitivity, the use of more resilient, damping occlusal materials and/or adjusting a less intimate occlusal contact of 10–100 microns when opposing a natural tooth or another implant is clinically recommended [5].

A final aspect in dental tooth compliance, relevant to any type of restorative procedure is the stiffness of the tooth components. While the PDL offers viscoelastic, hydrodynamic damping properties at lower, physical masticatory loading, the elasticity of the supporting tooth structure for a restoration plays an important role at higher loads. Such higher loads might even exceed the physiological range and the tooth-restoration compartment need to withstand parafunctional loads during bruxing or clenching. The elasticity of the supporting tissue is thus tailoring the restoration design. Due to the high mineral content of 86 vol% Hydroxyapatite in human enamel, the elastic modulus is reported in the range of approximately 80–100 GPa [17]. In contrast, Dentin is less mineralized, containing only 45 vol% anorganic hydroxyapatite interconnected with 30 vol % fibrous organic collagens. Dentin is hence reported to exhibit an elastic modulus of approximately 15–20 GPa [18]. Such data need to be handled with care, as highly varying data can be found in literature, mainly due to age, location, and methodological approach to natural human teeth. Figure 5.24 shows an example of a human tooth that gives rise to the natural variations in composition and dimension. Once restoration is prepared in dentin, however, a more compliant support is expected, compared to underlying enamel.

5.2   Engineering Basics

Every single tooth has a unique shape and dimension, and once it comes to removal of carious tissue and preparation of a cavity, the shape still remains singular in each case. External loading on such an undefined structural component is hence not predictable. In order to enable and ensure a safe and mechanically stable design of a dental prosthesis, certain preparation guidelines are already manifested for years in restorative dentistry and hold for the clinical success. However, with development of new materials, technologies, and treatment procedures, those established guidelines might be subjected to continuous reappraisal of mechanical and clinical validity. In this context, especially handling modern ceramic materials requires a sound knowledge of engineering basics in order to understand and validate the individual treatment strategy.

5.2.1   Principal Loading Directions

When load is applied on a structural component—such as teeth—the reaction is related to microstructural displacement and deformation. Such deformation can be either reversible or nonreversible, in the way that we commonly distinguish elastic and plastic material response. With increasing load, most materials respond in an elastic, reversible way, followed by a nonreversible, plastic deformation. This frame of mechanical behavior can be extended by the time component. Once a material shows a time-dependent, retarded behavior, that is called a viscoelastic or viscoplastic response, in contrast to a time-independent material response.

Regarding dental restorations, a plastic or even viscoelastic material response is not desirable and hence narrows down our focus to purely elastic, time-independent mechanical behavior [19]. The mechanical behavior of structural materials is commonly approached by stress–strain experiments under certain loading conditions.

External forces or moments are initially applied on a structural component but more important is the stress that is created in the component. So the external load F divided by the area under load A defines the stress σ. The loading direction onto the area further distinguishes the type of stress. Once the force is applied perpendicular to the area, we call that a normal stress σ, once the force is oriented parallel to the area this is termed shear stress τ.

$$\sigma = \frac{F_\perp}{A} \tag{5.1}$$

$$\tau = \frac{F_\parallel}{A} \tag{5.2}$$

In reality, normal and shear stresses act simultaneously and contribute to the overall stress state.

The response of a component to external stress is commonly expressed by local displacements in the microstructure resulting in deformation of the body. Such dimensional changes are termed strains ε. We analogously to the stress direction distinguish normal strains ε and shear strains γ. While normal strains are characterized by changes in length, shear deformations are described by the shear angle (compare Fig. 5.5).

In the linear-elastic range of material response, the normal stress σ is related to the normal strain ε, via the material constant E, called Young's or elastic modulus.

$$\sigma = E \cdot \varepsilon \tag{5.3}$$

This relationship is called the Hooke's law and characterizes the stiffness of a material in terms of stiffer behavior at higher elastic moduli. This law, however, is only valid for uniaxial loading and small strains. The analogous relationship can be derived for shear loadings. The shear modulus G, thereby relates the shear stress τ to the shear strain γ.

$$\tau = G \cdot \gamma \tag{5.4}$$

In the same way, the shear modulus G characterizes the stiffness of a material under shear conditions. The dimensional change in one direction however triggers a compensation in the transversal direction, e.g., as a material is elongated under tension, it contracts in the perpendicular direction. Such contractions are expressed by the Poisson's ratio ν. The Poisson's ratio further

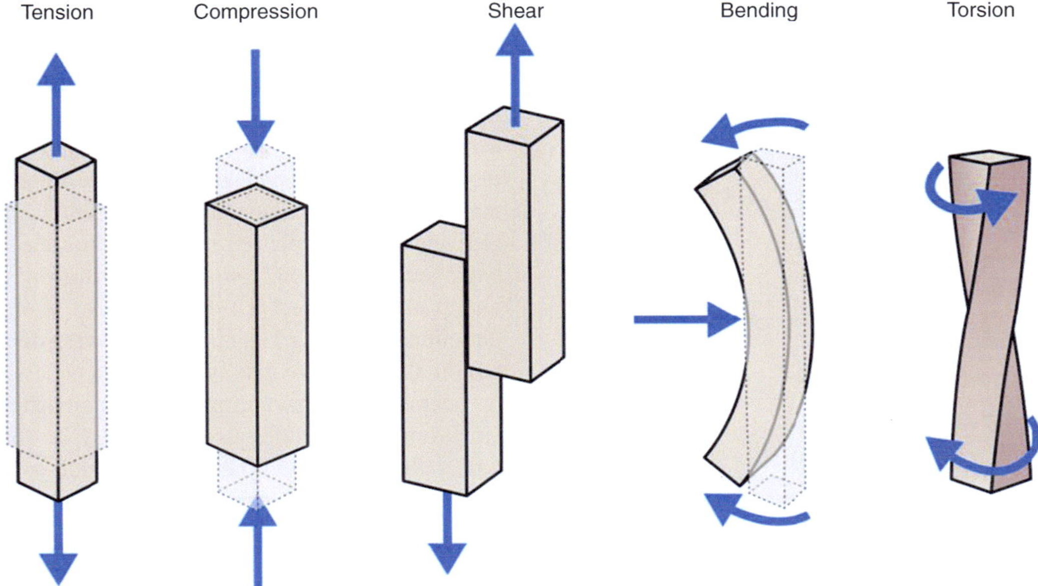

Fig. 5.5 Principal loading directions on a structural component

relates the elastic modulus in uniaxial loading with the shear modulus in shear loading.

$$G = \frac{E}{2(1+v)} \qquad (5.5)$$

In principle, five major kinds of loading are distinguishable: tension, compression, flexure, shear, and torsion. Figure 5.5 schematically illustrates the respective loading directions.

Uniaxial stress applied in tensile direction causes elongation of a component. Vice versa, a material reacts with contraction under uniaxial compressive stress. Tangentially applied shear stress causes deformation in terms of internal sliding of structural elements. Torsion is characterized by twisting of a component upon torque moments.

Among principal loading directions, special attention is drawn to a component under bending conditions. The external bending moment thereby combines elongation on the tensile side with contraction on the compressive side of a component. A neutral plane within the body accounts for neither tension nor compression and Fig. 5.6 illustrates the stress profile in bending configuration.

Figure 5.6b shows the shear forces are constant over the beam, however, counteracting each other and being zero under the central load roller. In 4-point bending, the shear forces are acting only in the outer regions between the upper and the lower load rollers, being zero in the central region between the upper load rollers. The maximum bending moment ($M_{max} = FL/4$), however, is active under the central load roller (in 3-point bending, see Fig. 5.6c or constantly distributed between the upper load rollers (in 4-point bending). This zone is free of shear stress and hence under pure bending conditions. As moments have to be in equilibrium ($\Sigma M = 0$), a reactive moment of inertia, I, has to counteract the bending moment. This moment is reflecting the geometry of the component under load and is quantifying the cross section (also referred to as shape factor or section modulus). Finally, the maximum bending stress in a beam is defined by the ratio of $\sigma_{max} = M/I$ [20, 21]. With the section modulus of $I = wb^2/6$ for rectangular specimens (w: width; b: thickness), we end up with:

$$\sigma_{max} = \frac{M}{I} = \frac{3FL}{2wb^2} \qquad (5.6)$$

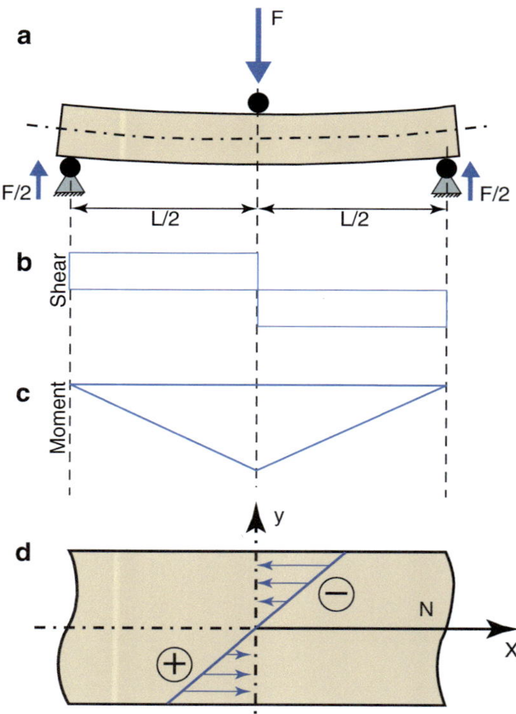

Fig. 5.6 A rectangular bend bar under 3-point bending conditions (**a**). The development of shear force (**b**) and bending moment (**c**) with its maximum under the central load roller as well as schematic of the stress distribution through the thickness of the bend bar (**d**) showing the regions under compression (−) and tension (+), with the neutral plane (N) separating both regions

the equation that is provided in ISO 6872 for calculation of flexural strength in a 3-point bending configuration [22].

Among the five loading cases, tension is the most critical scenario, especially for brittle, purely elastic materials. By reaching the ultimate strength level, a brittle ceramic would fracture upon tensile overloading in the maximum loaded volume. Even under compressive conditions, tensile stress will develop and account for failure. It is most unlikely that a ceramic body fails due to compressive stress. Even in bending conditions, the maximum tensile stress is located on the tensile side of a bending bar and failure is caused by tension. One of the main engineering principles with ceramics is hence to transform tensile into compressive loads by structural optimization.

Regarding dental prosthesis, we are able to identify all sorts of loading conditions, for example, tensile conditions at the adhesive interface in high c-factor configurations, in radial alignment at crown margins, or in stress concentrated regions at design notches (e.g. brigde connectors). Those principal loading configurations provide an idealized picture of the stress state. In engineering of dental prostheses, however, we would always expect a combination of loading directions, resulting in a cumulative stress distribution. Compressive load is very likely occurring on occlusal surfaces during biting or clenching. However, the resulting applied stress is commonly distributed as a bending type due to the restoration compliance and loading directions. A specific, compressive loading case is the Hertzian contact situation, in which an occlusal point contact is compressively loaded. As occlusion, in reality, is a lateral dynamic movement, it has been shown that Hertzian contacts are even overlaid by sliding, shear stresses [23]. Shear is also a very typical loading type, especially during chewing or bruxing. A shear component is always effective and contributes to the overall stress state as we do not have perpendicular loading to a normal plane, especially at dynamic contacts. Shear is effective, e.g., at adhesive interfaces or at cusp flanges. Bending is the most likely loading configuration on dental prosthesis with crowns under axial load or at connector regions in multi-span bridges. Bending is a typical loading case regarding the stiffness of root canal points. Torsion in contrast is certainly a type of loading that is related to an unphysiological loading or to screw torques upon implant treatment. More examples will be provided in the context of this chapter.

Externally applied load on a body, as shown in Fig. 5.5, always reveals a normal stress component as well as a shear stress component. Both stress types are overlaid but in diverging directions. This fact creates a complex relationship between tensile, compressive, and shear stresses when external loads are not purely unidirectional but highly individual. A simple design tool for understanding and estimating stresses, hence designing optimized dental prostheses, is the

Method of Shear Squares, that will be introduced in the next chapter.

5.2.2 "Thinking Tools After Nature" © by Prof. Mattheck

This chapter provides an introduction to simple structural optimization. As we learned the knowledge of different stress states according to principal loading direction, we now focus on design and shape optimization of structural components. Basically, this chapter summarizes a scientific research line of Prof. Mattheck and co-workers, experts in fracture mechanics on the one side and in tree mechanics on the other side. Situated at the Karlsruhe Institute of Technology, Germany, they investigated on fundamental mechanical behavior of trees and many other forms in nature, and therefrom derived rules of nature that can be biomimetically translated and used in engineering design and shape optimization. Prof. Mattheck published a series of clearly written, highly informative books, that are strongly recommended for further reading [21, 24, 25]. Here, we introduce some of Prof. Mattheck's basic concepts that can be easily applied to any issue related to engineering design, as we might use them in dental cavity preparation and construction of individual dental prosthesis. These concepts have even found their way to international standardization and can be accessed through ISO 18459: Biomimetics—Biomimetic structural optimization [26].

In classical structural optimization, the aim is to reduce stress concentration to a minimum and hence to allow for a homogeneous force flow and stress distribution upon external loading, exactly the aim that we are following when it comes to dental cavity preparation. ISO 18459 introduces several optimization tools, with the majority based on complex numeric simulations. On the basis of finite element analysis (FEA), the biomimetic approaches in Computer Aided Optimization (CAO), Computer Aided Internal Optimization (CAIO), or Soft Kill Option (SKO) are introduced. Much simpler, and not even relying on complex calculations, the "Method of

Tensile Triangles" (MTT) is further part of the standard, aiming for easy understanding and application.

5.2.2.1 The Method of Shear Squares (MSS)

Prior to any design optimization, however, we need to understand and estimate the stress state in a body. Assuming that external loading boundaries are known (which is rarely the case, as local chewing forces remain undefined and local loading directions on an occlusal surface are highly individual), we do not know how those forces are transduced through the body. Various natural tissue or synthetic replacement materials have varying stiffness and internal interfaces might account for local barriers in terms of load transfer. With principal stress consisting of a normal stress as well as of a shear stress component, it becomes mandatory to identify the weak links in a body and learn the lessons from fractography and how structural components fail under either normal or shear loading.

In engineering design, numerical approximations via CAO, CAIO, or SKO techniques will help to clearly identify the weak links and to reshape a component for minimum stress concentration. This, however, is not an appropriate solution, when dentists are treating patients and need to ad hoc decide how to prepare a cavity and how to design the restoration. Prof. Mattheck developed a simple tool that allows to establish a relationship between local tensile, compressive, and shear stress components. He termed his first thinking tool the "Method of Shear Squares" (MSS) [25]. This tool is based on directional considerations. Basically, shear stresses are built up when a body resists to any sliding movement. The shear component is maximized under an angle of 45° to the applied (normal) load [27]. Taking the shear loading case from Fig. 5.5, we can draw the directions of tensile or compressive forces. What is happening upon resistance, e.g., at an internal interface, is that we are facing internal tensile and compressive forces under 45° inclinations to the external load. The sum of the resistant forces can also be written as shear forces in longitudinal and transversal directions.

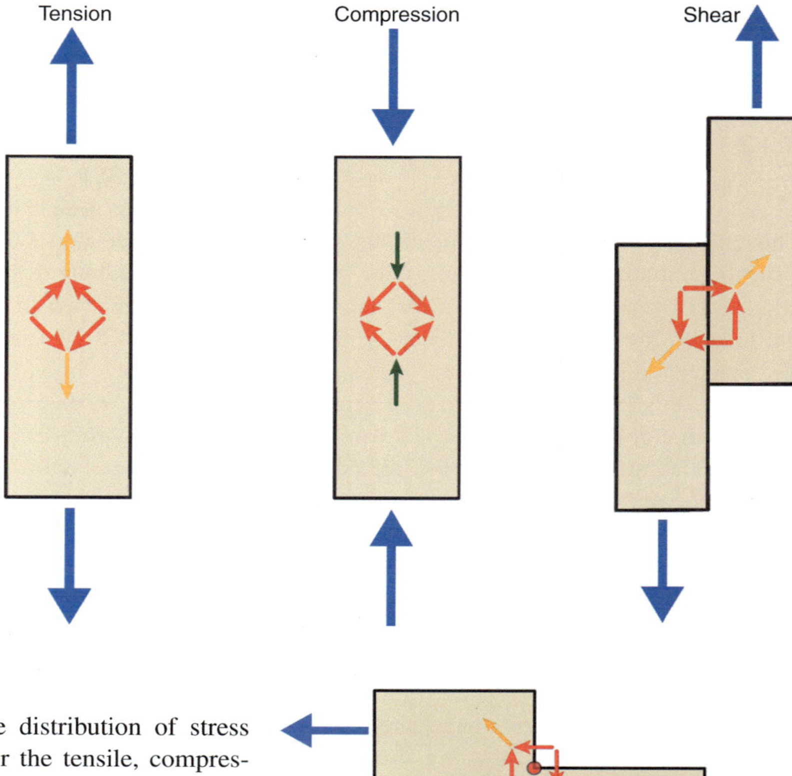

Fig. 5.7 Principal loading directions as outlined in Fig. 5.5 with respective shear squares. Tensile stress (yellow), compressive stress (green), and shear (red) components are labelled, indicating the stress state in a body under external load (blue) [25]

Figure 5.7 illustrates the distribution of stress upon external loading for the tensile, compressive, and shear loading conditions.

Beside the distribution and direction of stress in the bulk of a component, the contact of occlusal surfaces between the mandibular and maxillary dentition is of major importance to the stress transfer. Occlusal point contacts at cusp flanges can either be induced in normal direction (clenching) or under shear conditions (bruxing). In most cases, a mixture of normal and shear components is expected (compare Sect. 5.1.2). Upon knowledge of the respective loading contacts, the direction of a propagating crack can be estimated using shear squares. Occlusal point contacts are addressed in detail in Sect. 5.3.4.

5.2.2.2 The Method of Tensile Triangles (MTT)

The application of this technique to component edges brings us to the second thinking tool—the "Method of Tensile Triangles" (MTT), which offers simple guidance toward stress-reduced preparations. Figure 5.8 shows a rectangular corner in a random component under shear loading.

Fig. 5.8 Schematic illustration of the MSS. The notch is a critical location of stress concentration with tensile stress developing under 45° inclinations to the external load. A potential fracture plane (crack) might progress perpendicular to the tensile stress [24]

As the notch is under stress, we overlay our shear square and receive the resulting direction of the critical tensile stresses.

The level of stress concentration is thereby dependent on the size and shape of the notch, with decreasing stress at blunt notches and increasing stress at longer notches. The curvature is hence the design solution for reduction of notch stress concentration. This concept is certainly not new, but the MTT is extending this towards further reduction of notch stress in the direction of loading. Figure 5.9 shows a simple design solution for notch stress optimization.

Briefly, the MTT is biomimetically derived on the system of stem root junctions of trees and consists of adaptive triangle to ease notch stresses, as shown in Fig. 5.10.

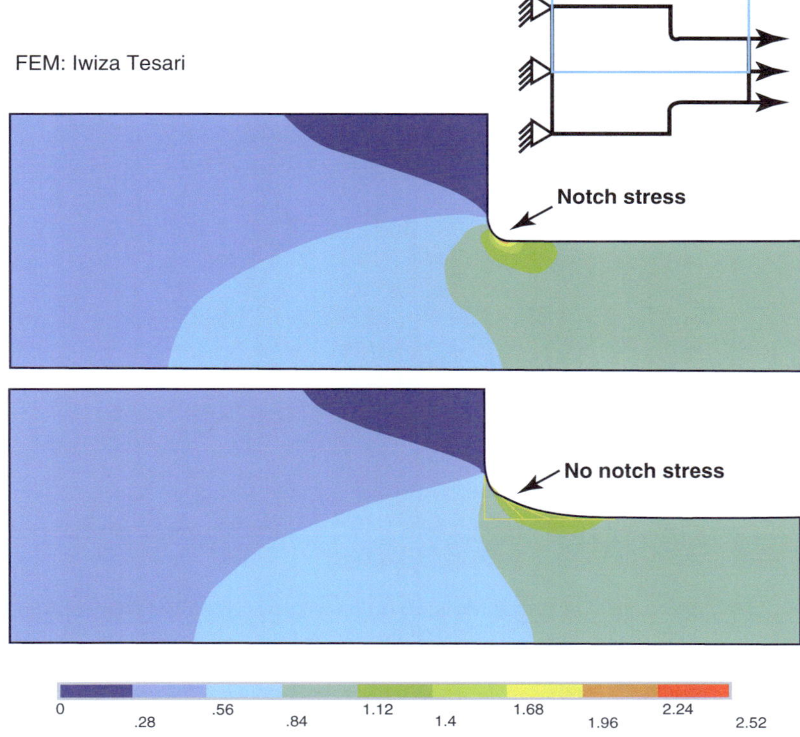

Fig. 5.9 FE model of a rectangular notch under external tensile loading. With increasing curvature in the loading direction, stress concentration can be minimized—with permission from the authors [25]

For uniaxial load cases, placing a tensile triangle contour in the notch, as shown in Fig. 5.9, is the maximum support. Multiaxial loading, however, might require overlaying tensile triangle arrangements in multiple directions. The notch effect is not just limited to structural components, but is even more effective on small surface or subsurface defects under tensile load, as further explained in Sect. 5.3.1.

5.2.2.3 The Biomimetic Principle of Whirl Toughening

Trees or wood consist of a fiber-like texture that allows for specific mechanical properties alongside as well as perpendicular to the alignments. Stiffness and elasticity are hence tailored by the anisotropic, hierarchical microstructure. When growing trees are under certain external loads that diverge from their target alignments, nature responds with creation of fiber kinking and twisting along a preferred shear plane. As slip or shear might be maximized under 45°, wood starts creating whirls in those highly loaded

regions [24]. The principle of whirl toughening in nature is further explained by Prof. Mattheck's "Method of Force Cones" (MFC) [28].

In principle, the human enamel is using the same toughening concept. The hierarchical structure of enamel is over wide-length scales characterized by aligned enamel prisms. Those parallel fiber bundles are radially oriented from the inner dentin to the outer occlusal surface. Occlusal forces in general act in the direction of the prisms and are thus an easy target for fracture. Nature has reinforced the enamel structure in highly loaded regions, as there are the occlusal cusp contacts or the stress concentrated fissure region. Summarized under the term "Hunter-Schreger-Bands," the orientation in those subsurface regions is characterized by interlaced and twisted (decussated) enamel prisms [29]. Figure 5.11 shows an example of this effective toughening mechanism in deeper enamel regions. It has been shown that the fracture toughness of enamel is potentially increasing in those regions, with a prominent R-curve

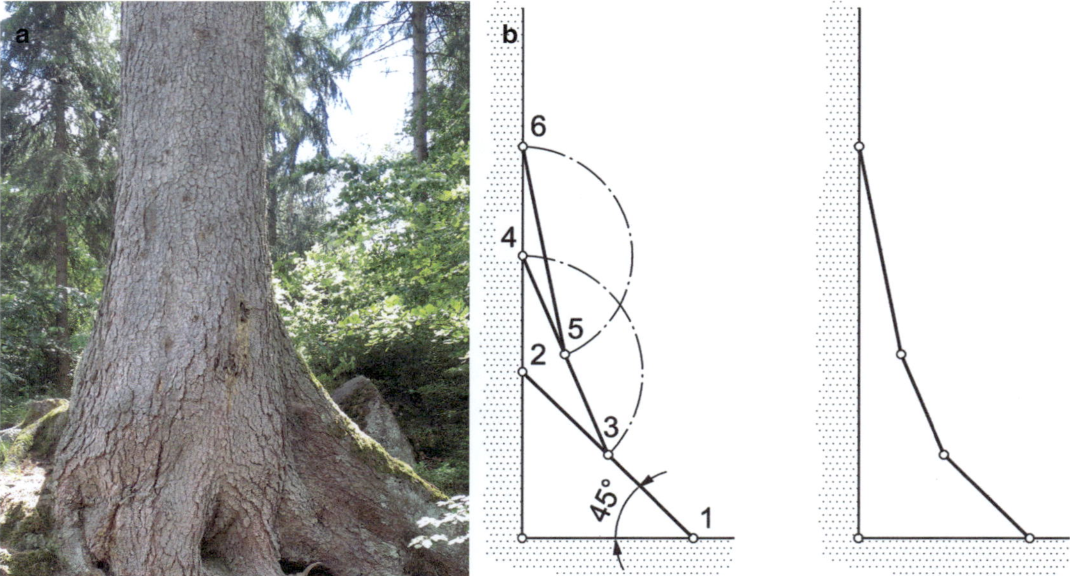

Fig. 5.10 The method of tensile triangles; (**a**) biomimetically derived from stem roots of a tree; (**b**) schematically applied on a rectangular notch, hence adapting a curvature with reinforcement triangles in the loading direction [26]

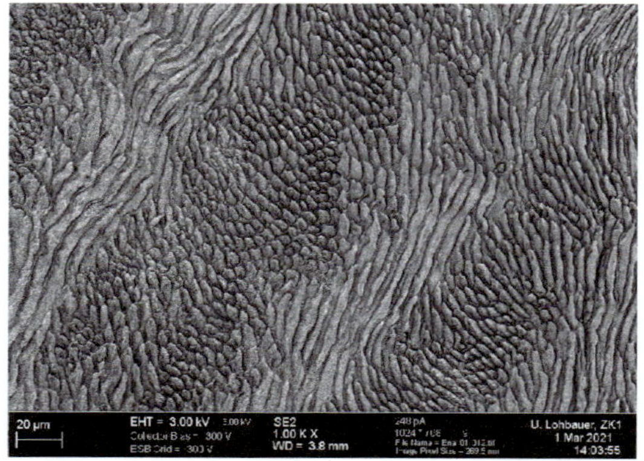

Fig. 5.11 Enamel prism decussation (Hunter-Schreger-Bands) acts as toughening mechanism in deeper enamel

effect rising from $K_{Ic} = 0.8$–1.5 MPam$^{0.5}$ in the outer to $K_{Ic} = 4.4$ MPam$^{0.5}$ in the inner region of human enamel [30]. Enamel decussation is also likely to act as a toughening mechanism in stress concentrated regions such as under occlusal contacts or in deep fissures.

5.2.2.4 Thinking Tools and the Natural Tooth

The validity of the MSS and MTT tools has conclusively been shown to hold for tree mechanics, but there is further extension and validity for any natural principle of growth and resistance. As this book is addressed to dentists and dental scientists, we will apply those concepts to a molar tooth. Figure 5.12 shows the application of MSS and MTT in various locations onto the geometry of a natural tooth. When a tooth becomes masticatory loaded, e.g., vertically load, several observations can be derived:

1. Occlusal contacts are loaded under compression (Hertzian point contact, see also Figs. 5.23 and 5.24). Further description of local stress distribution is provided in Sect. 5.3.4. A potential crack in return would propagate perpendicular to the tensile stress. A clinical example is the chipping of an occlusal

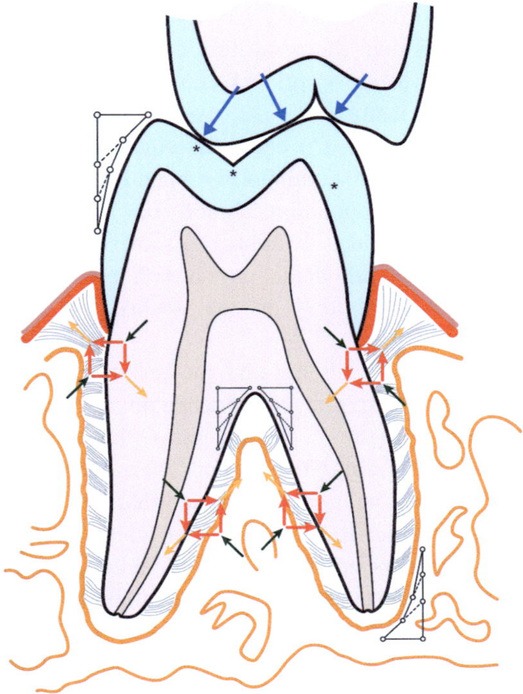

Fig. 5.12 Molar teeth in occlusal contact (point contacts are indicated with blue arrows). Applications of MSS and MTT show the principles of stress transfer. The mechanism of enamel toughening (whirl concept) is shown to act as "shear killer" in stress concentrated regions and deeper enamel layers

cusp under Hertzian contact, as shown in Fig. 5.25 [31].

2. The occlusal loading on two opposing cusp flanges creates stress concentration in deep fissures (notch effect). Initially compressive in nature, the stress concentration is perpendicular to the external load and a crack is expected to propagate vertically. A design optimization of the fissure region would include a larger notch radius as well as less inclined cusp flanges [32]. Further details can be found in Sect. 5.3.4.

3. The outer shape of the enamel crown follows the principles according to MTT in order to deflect and transfer occlusal stresses more homogeneously to the underlying bone.

4. The tooth root and the alveolar bone follows the shape proposed by the MTT, in order to minimize local stress concentrations arising from occlusal normal and shear forces.

5. The periodontal ligament (PDL) fiber bundles are oriented perpendicular to the applied load. While the alveolar crest fibers resist the forces in lateral shear direction, horizontal and mainly oblique fibers resist the tooth mobility against vertical, occlusal forces.

5.3 Applied Construction and Design

Every dentist has certainly been taught the principles of engineering design during their practical education. Based on former cavity classifications, e.g., according to Black, and intensive teaching of respective preparation guidelines, this training has led to a proper and safe engineering design for the majority of dental restorative treatments. However, with modern minimal invasive techniques and high-performance materials, those rigid preparation concepts might be obsolete and new approaches need to fill the gap. A sound understanding of preparation concept is hence the prerequisite of a stress-free, safe, and long-lasting design. This chapter is dedicated to some general and important cases in dental engineering design.

5.3.1 The Surface

Strength, resistance, friction, wear, or fatigue—the mechanical performance of restorative materials is highly dependent on the quality of the surface in occlusion.

The quality of a surface is characterized by the defect population induced during either manufacturing in the dental technician's lab, the

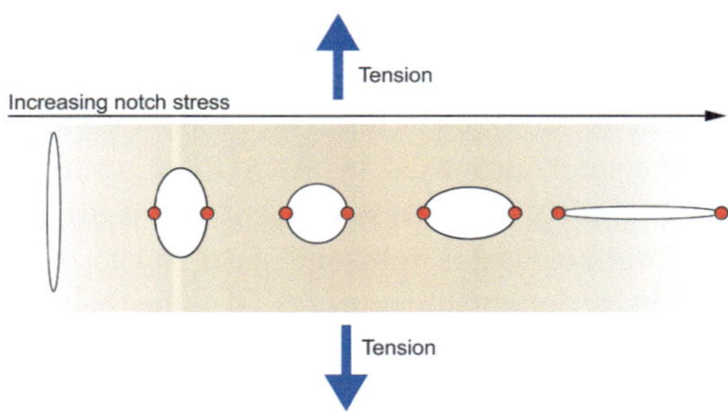

Fig. 5.13 Increasing notch effect of various defects under applied tensile stress

intraoral adjustment procedure during clinical placement, or during masticatory loading over the time in service. Depth, sharpness, location, and orientation in a loaded volume have an exponential influence on the resulting and expectable material strength performance, as this is related through the Irwin / Griffith concept of stress concentration (see Sect. 3.2). Figure 5.13 highlights the influence of shape and orientation of a defect (here: flaw/pore) to the applied stress. The notch effect is maximized when a sharp flaw is oriented perpendicular to the applied stress.

As we know from Fig. 5.6, the maximum effective moment in a rectangular specimen under bending conditions is located directly under the central load roller. This central region on the bottom side of the specimen is under maximum tensile stress and a fracture is most likely originated therein. Defects are hence most critical once located in this region, amplified by sharpness and orientation perpendicular to the tensile loading direction, as illustrated in Fig. 5.14.

According to Irwin, it becomes evident that the deepest defect is responsible for fracture initiation. Such defect populations on a ceramic surface are commonly measured by the roughness parameter Rz (mean roughness depth; in contrast to the average roughness (Ra)) as only this algorithm takes the complete vertical distance between the lowest valleys and the highest peaks into account and do not just average on mean roughness.

The surface of a dental restoration is adjusted with rotational diamond burs and subsequently polished using rotational diamond-in-silicone polishing instruments. As the intraoral adjustment procedure is a practical sequence of consecutive use of continuously finer instruments, the defect population should be thoroughly removed. Figure 5.15 however, shows an example of a fractured dental crown with remnants of the coarse grinding on the occlusal stressed surface.

Rotational grinding and the resulting defect depth have a significant influence on mechanical strength. Figure 5.16 illustrates the relation between mean roughness depth Rz and the measured biaxial strength of a dental lithiumdisilicate glass-ceramic. Red, yellow, and white labelled diamond burs are accounting for consecutively reduced coarseness. The flexural strength of the glass-ceramic exponentially increased with a decreasing Rz. Additional polishing is reducing the mean roughness depth Rz below 0.5 μm. In turn, the strength increased from 220 MPa (coarse ground surface, $Rz = 5.6$ μm) to 550 MPa (polished surface, $Rz = 0.5$ μm), a potential increase of 250%! A smoother surface and a lower defect population are thus the decisive determinants for preserving maximum strength of restorative materials.

Preparation design is guided to ensure the maximum surface quality in highly stressed regions of a prosthesis. Such regions are, e.g., the occlusal contact points (unfortunately those points are dedicated to intraoral adjustments) or at the gingiva side of bridge connectors.

Surface roughness is not just the result of intraoral adjustment procedures, but is very likely to develop during years of clinical service. A patient is exposed to mastication and occlusion. Physiological forces or para-functional overloads during bruxing or clenching accelerate the surface degradation and induce defects in the highly stressed occlusal regions. Figure 5.17 shows the occlusal surface of a posterior glass-ceramic crown on tooth #37 and from an anterior crown on tooth #41, both after 3 years in service.

The practical consequence for proper engineering design and clinical lifetime extension is

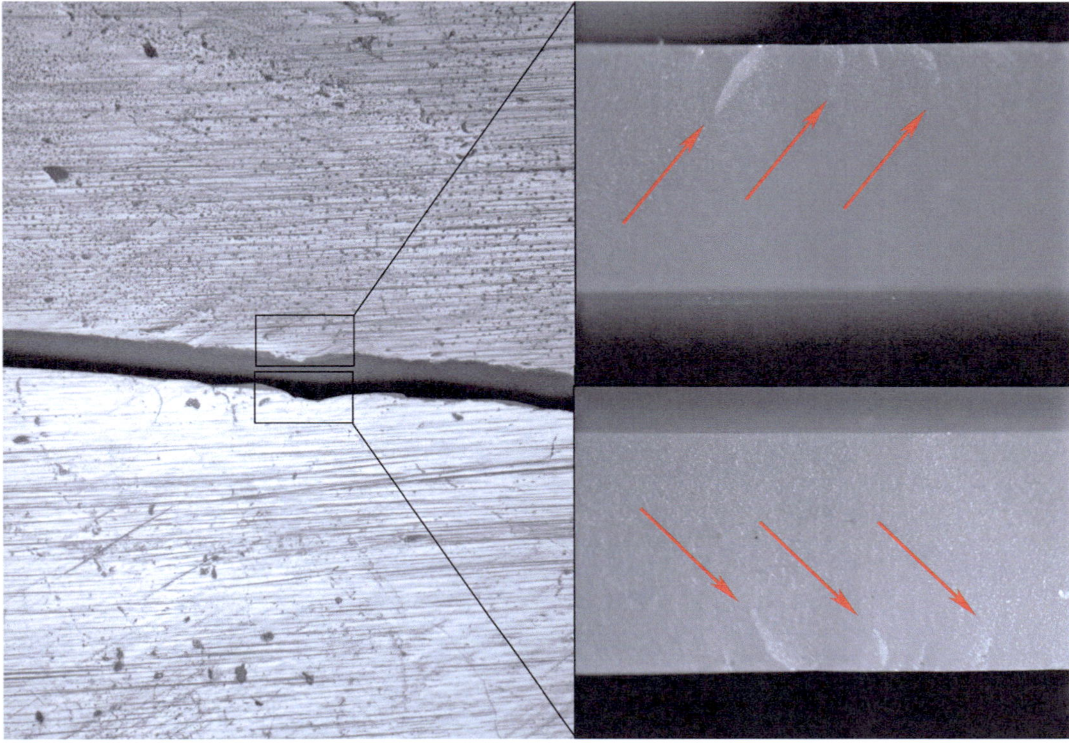

Fig. 5.14 A ceramic surface finished with rotational diamond burs in a direction perpendicular to the applied stress. The cross-sectional view shows extensions of deeper cracks into the specimen volume (red arrows)

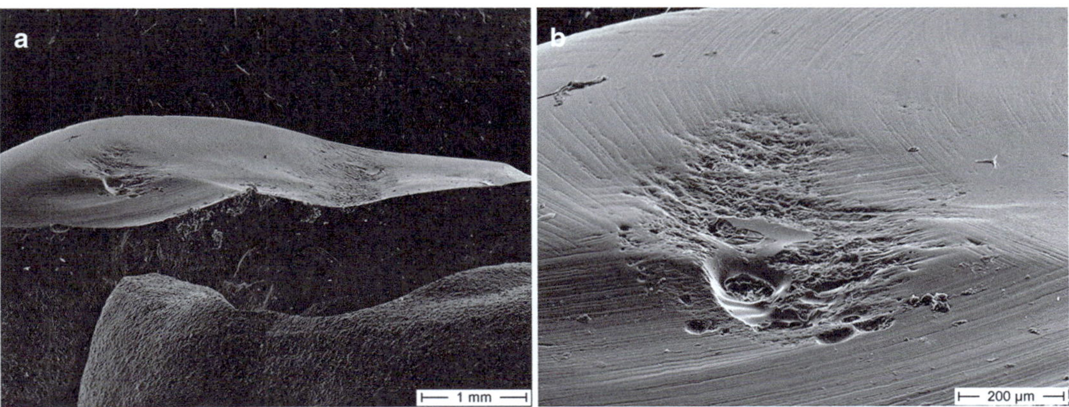

Fig. 5.15 Fractured posterior crown on tooth #37 (**a**). Coarse grinding defects are observable as well as incomplete polishing of the occlusal surface (**b**). The consecutive polishing sequence has not been followed

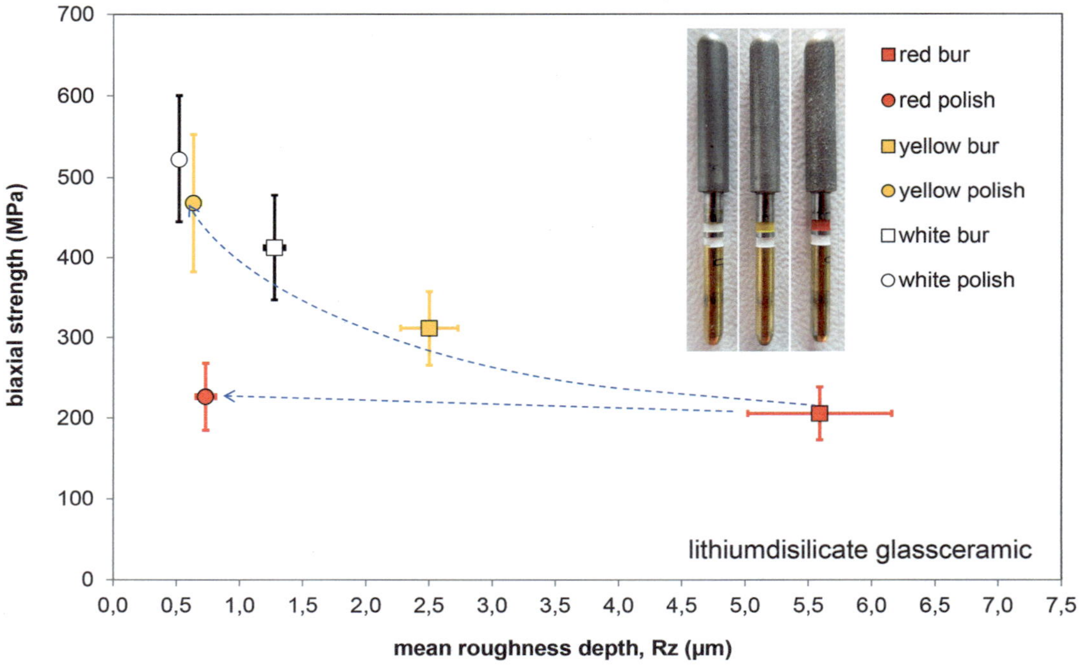

Fig. 5.16 Mean roughness depth (*Rz*) versus biaxial strength of a dental lithiumdisilicate glass-ceramic. The strength development upon a consecutive polishing sequence versus the direct polishing of an initially coarse ground surface is shown

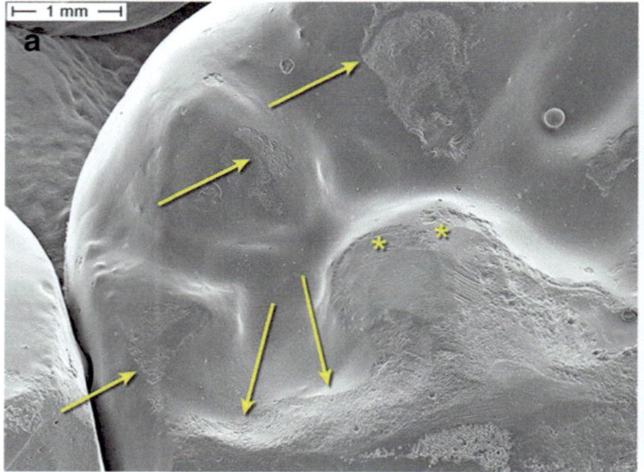
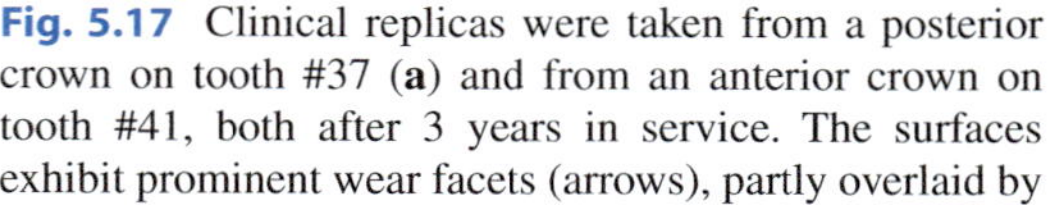
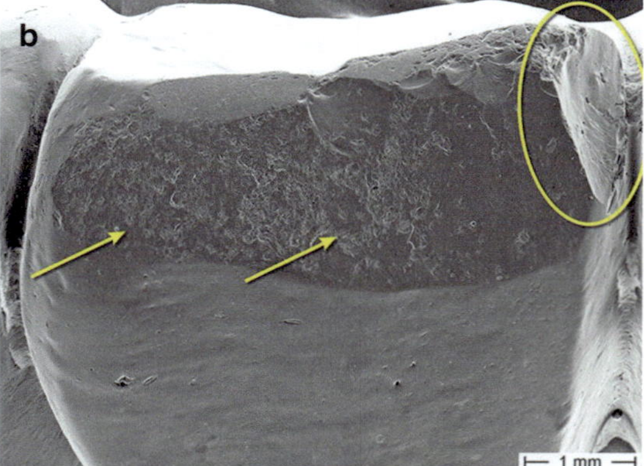

Fig. 5.17 Clinical replicas were taken from a posterior crown on tooth #37 (**a**) and from an anterior crown on tooth #41, both after 3 years in service. The surfaces exhibit prominent wear facets (arrows), partly overlaid by initial grinding damage (asterisks). The wear damage led to growth of defects, leading to incisal fracture (**b**; yellow circle)

related to a thorough preventive polishing of critical regions during dental recall sessions.

5.3.2   The Angles

Removal of caries and the preparation of a cavity, leading to the construction of a replacement filling has already been classified by G. V. Black back over 100 years ago. He created five classes of typical cavity designs and derived specific preparation guidelines according to established engineering principles. About 50 years ago, when adhesive dentistry broadly conquered the dental world and hence allowed for adhesive, support of joints, Black's concept step by step diminished as minimal invasive dentistry took over.

However, still the main prosthetic replacement strategy employs brittle ceramics such as lithiumsilicate glass-ceramics or polycrystalline zirconia. Along with the brittleness of restorative materials, the old preparation guidelines are still partly valid or even modified in a complex way. As simple as it is, a brittle material reacts extremely resistant against all types of compressive loading but is increasingly sensitive against shear, bending, or tensile external stress. Type of stress concentration, overloading, or excessive deflection has to be avoided. It becomes clear that minimum wall thickness of a restoration has to be preserved as well as blunted notches and edges are desirable wherever a cavity needs preparation and replacement with brittle ceramics. The classical site for such stress concentration is the bottom of a cavity preparation. The benefit of blunting those notches has been shown in elaborative finite element studies [33] or simply shown by application of the MTT [25]. Other than the tensile tringle that is shown in Fig. 5.18, the stress distribution effective at the bottom of a cavity, however, is of multiaxial nature and we need to extend the MTT in two dimensions.

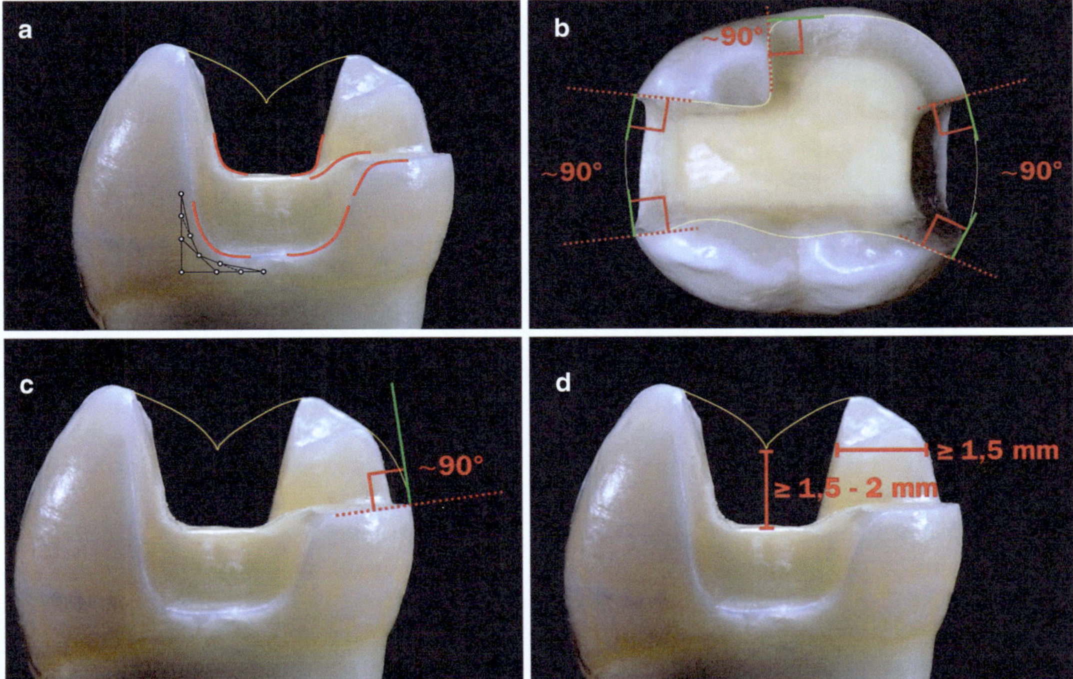

Fig. 5.18 Clinical preparation guidelines for a posterior single tooth replacement (Black class II cavity). The preparation of rounded internal angles (indicated by the MTT) is recommended (**a**) as well as preparation of external right angles (**b** and **c**). The preservation of minimum wall thickness (here: 1.5 mm under the central fissure or in cusp extension) is mandatory for a stiff and resistant absorption of occlusal forces (**d**) (images by courtesy of Priv-Doz. J. I. Zorzin, Erlangen, Germany)

Figure 5.18 shows a typical class II cavity on a molar tooth. Figure 5.18a shows ideal internally rounded angles, here simply evidenced by the overlaid MTT. We modified the MTT for a biaxial stress state in order to counteract vertical as well as horizontal forces. When it comes to external angles, however, the game, however, ends in tie, as enamel is a brittle material, too. As Fig. 5.18b shows, none of both, neither the ceramic nor the enamel should be forced in a sharp angle, resulting in a preparation window of 60°–90° angles. Of course, the occlusal surface is a specific case as the cusp inclination forces a divergent angle, otherwise, the inlay would not fit. Once the occlusal interface between restoration and enamel is close to the antagonist contact region, a full removal and replacement of the cusp is recommended.

The minimum thickness of a restoration is a critical aspect, as the majority of clinical fractured restorations are underrunning those recommendations. We learned the compliance of the natural tooth tissue (see Sect. 5.1.3) with dentin offering an elastic modulus of approximately 15–20 GPa. This compared to elastic properties of lithiumsilicates ($E = 100$ GPa) or zirconia ($E = 200$ GPa) makes clear that the underlying dentin is only a weak support and most of the occlusal load needs to be absorbed by the restoration itself [34]. As a result of reduced thickness, a substantial bending moment under occlusal contact is applied to the restoration, leading to fractures that emanating from the bottom side of the restoration [35]. A principle, experimental study on cracking in bilayer ceramics on low compliant substrates further elucidates the underlying principles, as radial cracking starts beneath the loading contact at the interface to the low compliant support, where maximum flexural tension occurs [36]. In a practical context, the minimum dimensions might be followed upon preparation, but this criterion could easily be failed after intraoral adjustment at critical, occlusal contacts. In order to get a feeling of the practical implications, a numeric study analyzed the occlusal crack initiation load with increasing crown thickness [37]. For a variety of contemporary restorative materials, the authors found a 100% increase in fracture resistance by increasing the material thickness from 0.7 to 1.3 mm.

On the basis of the outlined preparation guidelines, working with indirect ceramic replacements is not a truely minimal invasive alternative and as long as it possible, a direct, minimal invasive resin composite filling should be preferred.

5.3.3 The Margins

The quality of margins is a central concern in engineering design, especially when using brittle ceramics. Today's ceramic restorations are to an increasing extent subtractively manufactured via CAD/CAM processing. We learned that surface grinding has a damaging effect on the resulting defect population by introducing deep surface or even subsurface cracks into the restoration (see Fig. 5.14). All regions under tensile stress, amplified at low material thickness or sharp angles are prone to fracture when coinciding with such defects. The cervical margins of a crown or bridge are key locations as well as sharp transitions at inlay margins. Figure 5.19 shows an example of a CAD/CAM manufactured, experimental crown dome in higher magnification.

The fracture resistance of such a region is hence important for the overall integrity of a restoration. Figure 4.11e, f and i, j show examples of marginal crown fractures. This type of failure is a common clinical fracture mode, often observed during initial placement of a restoration [38, 39]. A combined clinical and experimental research investigated on this failure type and found influences from hydrolytically expanding cements and tapered crown preparations leading to build-up of hoop stresses in the marginal region [40]. The authors developed an experimental test routine to closely simulate this clinical fracture mode. The tangential normal stress build-up in the marginal region is schematically shown in Fig. 5.20. Based on a presumed hoop stress fracture mode, we derived a sphero-cylindrical model for dental crowns in order to investigate on the influencing factors [41]. The experimental findings were supported by finite element modelling as well as retrospective fractography. Figure 5.21

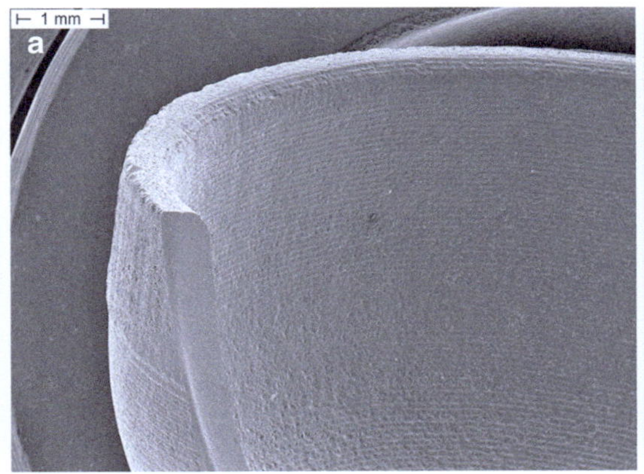

Fig. 5.19 Margin quality of a CAD/CAM manufactured crown analogon (dome shape). The margin defects are created upon fine rotational machining of a chamfer preparation using a feldspathic ceramic (**a**). A higher magnification shows the severity of sharp defects at the outer face of the dome as well as the grinding grooves on the whole surface (**b**; arrows). The MTT indicates the rounded shoulder margins

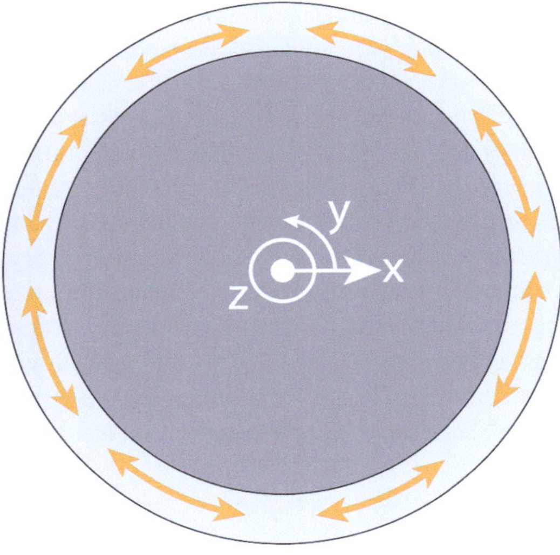

Fig. 5.20 Schematic drawing of the tangential "hoop" stress component, transferred into normal tensile stresses [41]

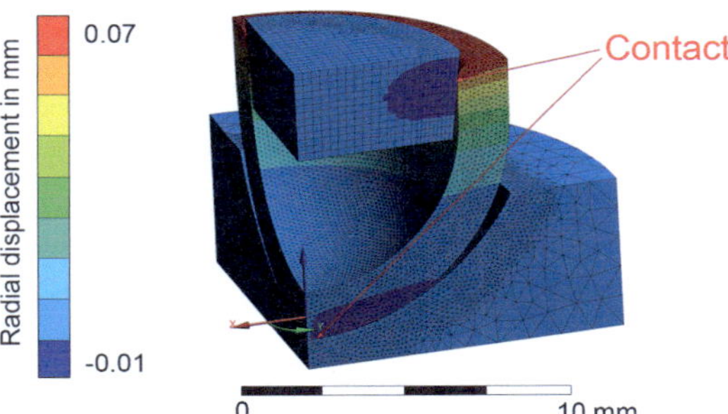

Fig. 5.21 Test setup of the "hoop-strength" test with dome-like ceramic crown analogons radially loaded to fracture using a tapered steel plunger [41]

shows the simulated setup of this "hoop-strength" test [41].

We compared different materials at different marginal thicknesses and concluded that marginal strength is greater for stronger and tougher ceramics and that thicker margins resist the hoop stress component to a higher degree compared to thin margins. Most interestingly, however, is the influence of CAD/CAM machining defects on marginal strength. The machining damage was found more severe at outer edges of the rim due to sharp angle with the surface (see Fig. 5.19b). The impact of machining defects on fracture initiation process is especially prominent for thin structures (here: 0.65 mm) with decreasing impact on thick margins (here: 1.65 mm). As per previous argumentation (see Sect. 5.3.1), the role of polishing or glace firing must not be underestimated for maximum strength preservation.

5.3.4 The Crown

The classic prosthetic replacement type is the single tooth full-coverage crown. This type of restoration was manufactured over decades with a metal core that was veneered with an esthetic, translucent feldspathic ceramic layer. Within the last two decades, the metal support was progressively replaced by ceramic core materials. Lithiumsilicate glass-ceramics and zirconia are the materials of choice for today's metal-free prosthetic treatments. As with increasing esthetic demands, the question still remained unsolved of how to create the best natural appearance. Veneering of the ceramic core materials is still a treatment option but with development of translucent and multilayer shaded zirconia, the trend guides toward monolithic restorations. CAD/CAM manufacturing seems to become the preferred processing route as an efficient and economic tool in the digital processing chain.

With transition from metal to all-ceramic single-tooth crowns, several design issues needed to be adapted to the brittle nature and risk against spontaneous fracture of the latter one. It turned out that preparation guidelines that held for formerly cemented metal-veneered crowns could not be simply transferred to adhesively luted, all-ceramic crowns and new construction concepts became essential. Regarding the single tooth molar crown, the design concept involved the occlusal curvatures on cusps and fissures as well as occlusal thickness and the inner core preparation. When considering veneered all-ceramic restorations, the thickness ratio between core and veneer plays a dominant role for a safe construction design. Finally, the preparation of margins is an important aspect of a load-resistant stress transfer.

A series of experimental and numerical studies have investigated on the influence of the occlusal curvature on the fracture resistance of all-ceramic single-tooth crowns [32, 37, 42, 43]. The notch angle in the central mesiodistal fissure is a target design parameter as well as the cusp inclination angle.

Finite element modelling is a useful technique toward stress analysis in a complex compartment as a single tooth crown. Figure 5.22 shows the distribution of maximum principal stress when a tooth contour is under occlusal loading.

The numerical simulation provides a detailed picture of the distribution of a specific stress state in local resolution and easily indicates stress concentrations at occlusal contacts and further impacts on the stress state in deep fissures. Based on stress concentrations, the expectance of likely fracture planes is guiding the construction design. A numeric simulation study investigated the stress distribution in occlusal fissures with varying cusp angles between 50° and 70° to the vertical axis and different fissure morphologies regarding notch sharpness [32]. This study presented a flat

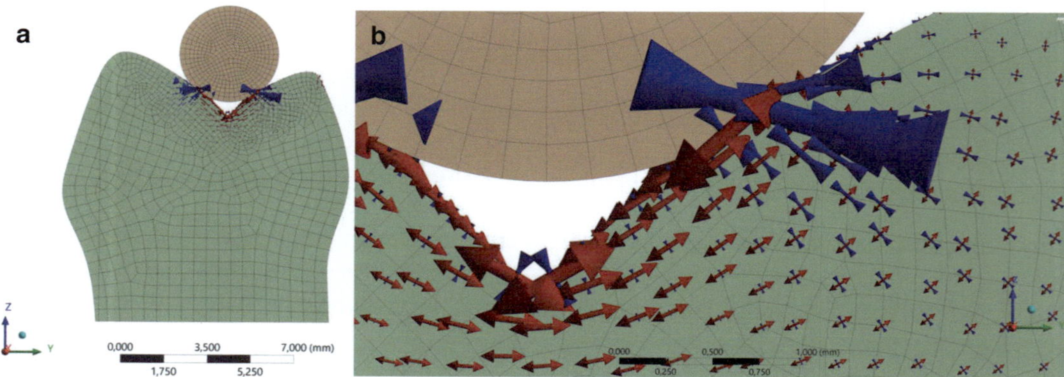

Fig. 5.22 3D FE model of occlusally loaded posterior crown (**a**). The tooth is loaded with a sphere in three-point contact and the inset (**b**) shows the direction of the principal stress vectors in the fissure region und under cusp contact points (first principal stress: red; third principal stress: blue; images by courtesy of H. Völkl, KTmfk, Erlangen, Germany)

curvature fissure morphology (reduced stress concentration) to better resist fracture under occlusal load. The same research group extended their studies to investigate on the influence of the cusp angles and material thickness [37]. They recommended a rounded occlusal notch (fissure), flat cusp angles (70°), and medium thickness (1.5 mm) as the optimum in terms of tooth preservation and fracture resistance. Preparations for using high-performance materials, such as zirconia, allow for reduced thickness (1.0 mm) and steeper cusp angles (60°). Adaptaion of cusp inclination angles are limited, as the fissure morphology is important for food crunching and transport and too flat cusp geometries are restraining dynamic occlusion [42]. A medium, buccolingual inclination of 60° to the vertical axis is recommended. The occlusal load effective on the cusp inclinations is further counteracted by compressive resistance at the proximal contacts.

Numerical studies commonly employ engineering boundaries and tend to simplify the situation to a certain extent. A sound molar tooth or a restored crown should have an intimate approximal contact with the neighboring mesial and distal tooth, which in turn prevents the lateral strain of a tooth under vertical, occlusal load. Hence, the stress concentration in a deep fissure is probably less than predicted and needs further attention. Friction at contact points has a further effect of the stress state in the occlusal fissure.

However, the overall distribution and qualitative prediction of normal or shear stresses can instantly be indicated by application of the MSS. Basically, a point contact under normal stress can be described as Hertzian contact while a contact under transversal, shear stress can be described as a sliding, dynamic contact [23]. Figure 5.23 shows the respective contact situations and the overlaid MSS. The direction of a propagating crack can easily be estimated.

The crack propagation under a normal loaded point contact, depends on the material thickness and the compliance of a supporting structure (e.g. due to dentin elasticity), leading to either a compressive or a bending stress state. In a thin plate, the bending moment becomes active while in a rather thick plate, the point contact is still a compressive, Hertzian type of stress. Under bending conditions, a crack would propagate from the bottom of the plate, while the compressive case would trigger shear cracks, inclined to the contact surface.

Figure 5.24 shows the practical implications of the above loading principles with clinically relevant fracture types. The notch effect of two

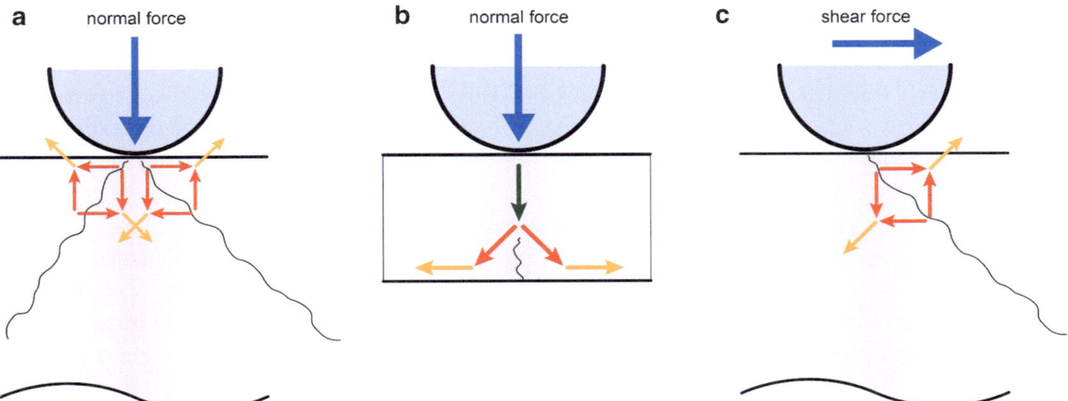

Fig. 5.23 Principle understanding of occlusal contact point mechanics under normal and shear forces showing the development of internal tensile stress and hence a likely direction of crack propagation upon overloading. While Hertzian contacts upon normal loading tend to initiate cone cracks starting at the contact zone (**a**), the contact in thin plates (as found is weakly supported or thin restorations) follows the bending configuration respective crack profiles (**b**). Under shear loading (**c**), the Hertzian pressure (e.g., upon severe bruxing) induces a cone type of crack that propagates ahead of the contact pressure zone

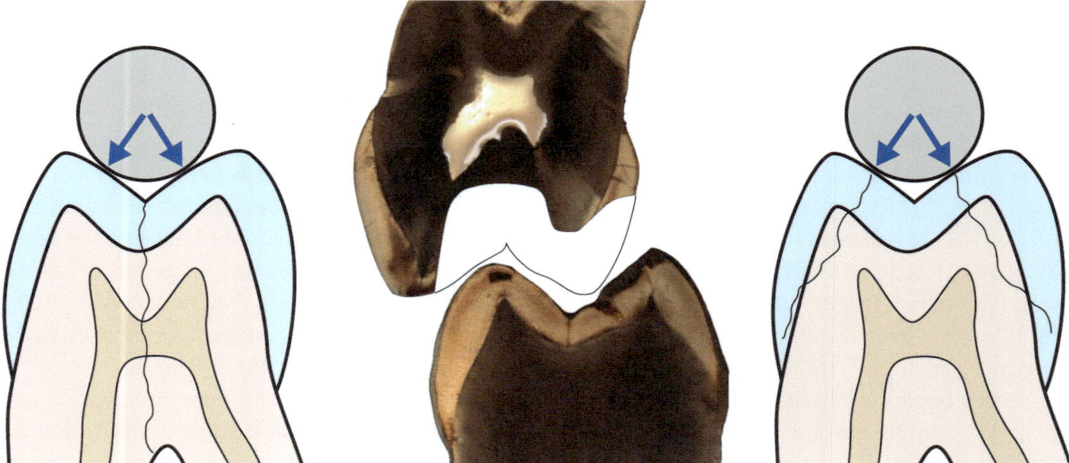

Fig. 5.24 Occlusal loading on first molars and schematic drawings of principle fracture types in the fissure region (left) and on cusp flanges (right)

simultaneous point contacts on cusp flanges is likely leading to fissure fracture, while the contact damage directly at occlusal contacts is rather producing cusp or chipping fractures.

The engineering design for posterior crowns was extended when using bilayered, veneered ceramic structures [44]. Numerical studies have investigated on the influence of the supporting core design on the fracture resistance of the veneer layer [43]. When using veneered structures, this research group found substantial stress concentration in the fissure region and recommended an anatoform, cusp supporting design of the underlying core material in order to prevent early fractures. Figure 4.11g, h shows an example of a fractured crown with missing anatoform support from the zirconia core. Figure 5.25 further shows an example of a fractured premolar crown (buccal chipping) starting from the cusp, progressing toward the oreveneer interface.

Another aspect regarding crown preparations is the margin design either at cervical or at incisal locations with the central purpose of providing stabilization against occlusal loads hence to resist fracture and to ensure a clinically acceptable marginal adaptation. Figure 5.26 draws different crown margin designs, of which only the chamfer and the rounded shoulder preparations are recommended for all-ceramic crowns.

It has been shown that marginal adaptation has a substantial impact on the fracture load on crowns upon cementation using, e.g., zinc phosphate cements [45]. Once the finish-line preparation allows for dry conditions (only supragingival preparations), an adhesive joint with the tooth core is preferable upon cementation as the load transfer is far more homogeneous through an adhesive layer. However, with clinically realistic margin openings of 50–100 μm, the adhesive layer is considerably stressed under occlusal loads. In order to minimize the stress concentration at the adhesive interface, the chamfer and the rounded shoulder are recommended for all-ceramic crown preparations [46], as shown in Fig. 5.26. The practical decision, however, is up to the treating dentist and is a balance between mechanical support and invasivity of the preparation. A rounded shoulder is more invasive compared to the chamfer preparation but provides better support under compression during occlusal loading. The tensile triangles indicate the benefit for a rounded axio-gingival preparation (see Fig. 5.26).

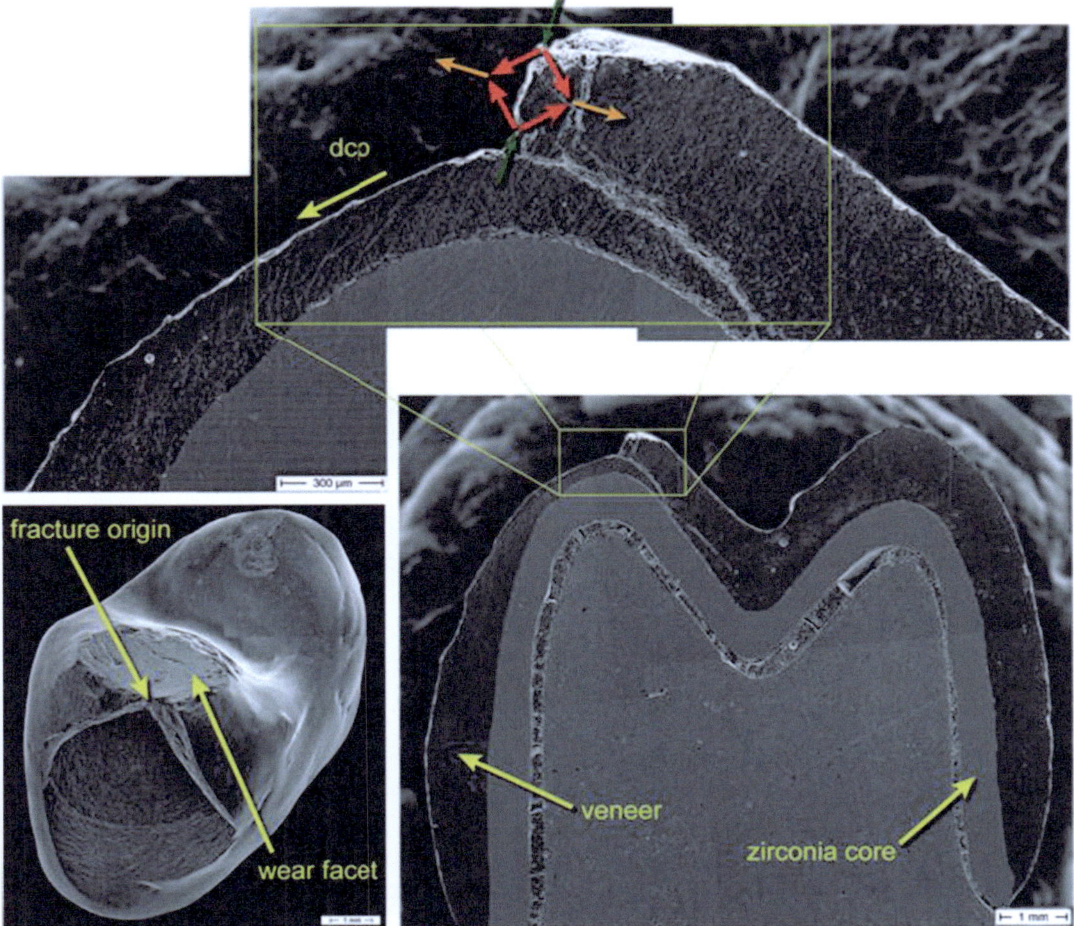

Fig. 5.25 A fracture case study shows occlusal loading on a cusp resulting in substantial chipping of the veneer layer. The dcp (direction of crack propagation) was identified perpendicular to the tensile stress component, as illustrated by the MSS [31]

The axial walls of a full-coverage crown are further stabilized by the proximal contacts. Intimate proximal contacts are essential to counteract shear stresses at the occlusal cusp surface with compression towards the neighboring teeth. Proximal contacts are point contacts between neighboring teeth in order to minimize the effective working area for caries. Upon restoration of two opposing proximal surfaces, this point contact might be re-engineered to a slightly flat area, hence reducing stress concentration. Figure 5.27 visually explains the mutual support between neighboring teeth with intimate proximal contacts.

5.3.5 The Bridge

A missing tooth can either be restored by a single-tooth implant or by a multi-unit prosthesis. A bridge hence requires at least one, typically two sound abutment teeth on which it

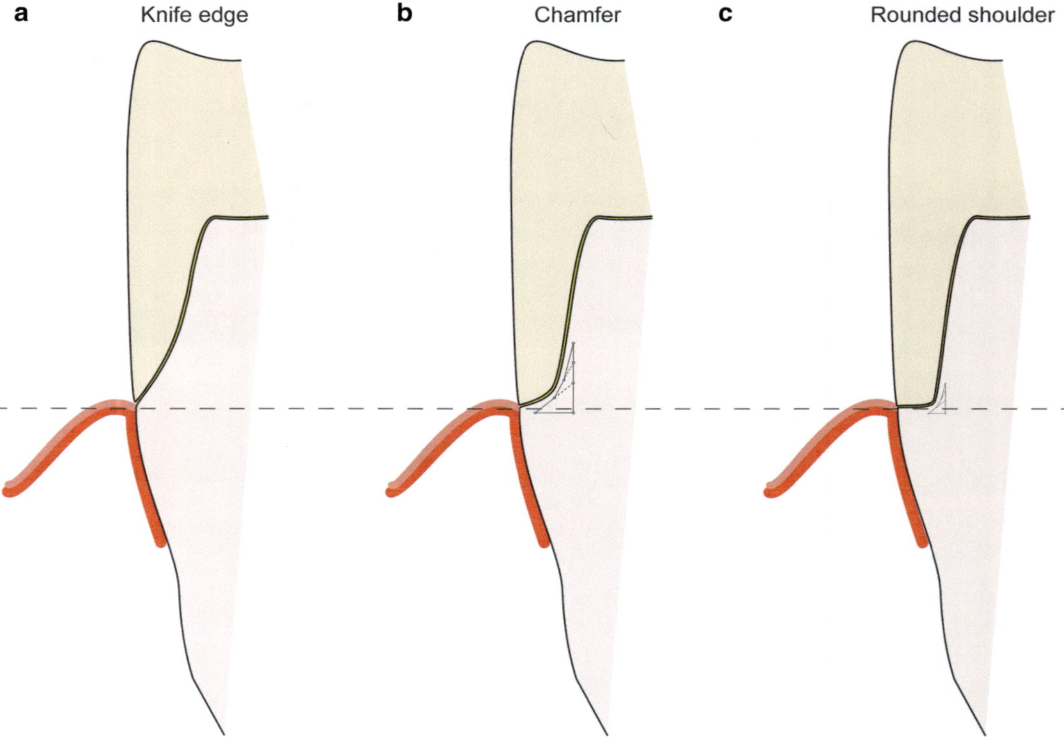

Fig. 5.26 Crown finish-line preparation: (**a**) knife-edge preparation; (**b**) chamfer preparation; (**c**) rounded shoulder preparation. Rounded axio-gingival angles are always recommended to reduce stress concentration (MTT overlay)

Fig. 5.27 Visualization of proximal contacts and mutual support and resistance against lateral strain upon occlusal loading

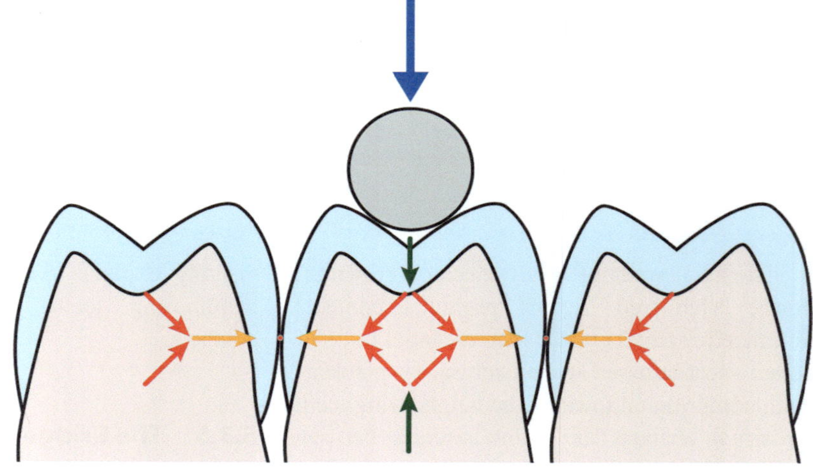

becomes attached. Highly individual in shape and design, a bridge generally consists of the abutment crowns and the pontic element (one or more units) that are jointed by the connectors. Figure 5.28 indicates a clinical fracture of a posterior three-unit bridge, manufactured of a veneered zirconia material. With the central aim to reconstruct oral function in harmonic occlusion, a bridge has to resist occlusal forces over a wide area and is hence a practical example for a bending configuration, as described in Sect. 5.2.1.

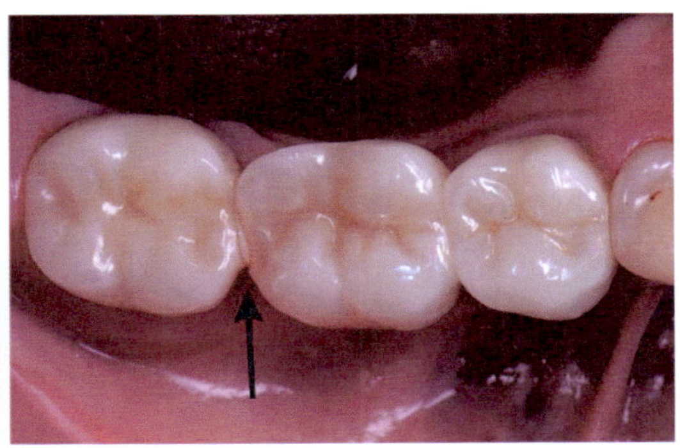

Fig. 5.28 Zirconia veneered, three-unit bridge with abutment crowns on teeth #45 and #47 and a pontic element on tooth #46. The arrow indicates a fracture in the connector region between tooth #46 and #47

The critical, weak links in this bridge "beam" are the connectors as the cross section is reduced in those regions. It has clinically been observed that this connector region is especially prone to fracture [47]. Figure 5.28 shows an example of a clinically fractured bridge connector. The fragile connector region under high bending loads has been addressed in several research studies, investigating on connector dimensions and design. Certain preparation guidelines were derived for specific locations.

Basically, we could think of simply simulating the bridge loading by using a continuous bending bar that is fixed at the length of the abutment teeth and vertically loaded on the central free pontic (in case of a three- or five-unit bridge) or on two free pontics (in case of a four-unit bridge), with the first one simulating a 3-point and the latter one simulating a 4-point bending configuration. Taking into account, that the bending stress is the ratio of the bending moment versus the moment of inertia ($\sigma = M/I$, see Sect. 5.2.2.1) and assuming that a connector has a circular or elliptical cross section, we replace the moment of inertia I to read [21]:

$$I = \frac{\pi w d^2}{32} \qquad (5.7)$$

This relation highlights the resistance against the bending moment to be related to a greater extent to the thickness d of a connector cross-section than to the width w.

Experimental studies have investigated on bridge connector dimensions. Based on minimum requirements for using, e.g., all-ceramic zirconia (3Y-TZP), a common standard of 9 mm² connector cross-sectional area has been indicated by the dental industry. This area however, can be composed of either variation in w/d ratio and/or in variations in shape.

Takuma et al. investigated on four-unit molar bridges made from zirconia [48]. With three connector sections under investigations, the w/d ratio of the elliptical shape at constant cross-sectional area of either 9 or 7 mm² was focused. They found fracture to occur mainly at the central connector at low thickness of the central connector ($w/d > 1$) and mixed with mesial or distal connectors at a greater thickness of the central connector ($w/d < 1$). They observed greater fracture forces with increasing cross-sectional area and increasing connector thickness, which is very much in common to the above consideration of the moment of inertia. The same group investigated on different shapes and dimensional ratio of zirconia three-unit bridge connectors, including isosceles or stretched triangle shapes with different orientations of the triangle to the vertically applied load [49]. They found significant differences among various designs at constant cross-sectional areas. No doubt, a greater cross-sectional area produced a greater resistance to fracture, but among w/d variations, the shape with maximum thickness offered the best resistance. Unfortunately, this was just shown under vertical loading while an incisor bridge is commonly exposed to a substantial shear loading. Figure 5.29a shows a connector fracture of a five-unit zirconia bridge with a sufficient cross-sectional area of 11.2 mm² but an unfavorable design as the flat side of the triangle limb is placed under compression and is not reinforcing the tension side. Figure 5.29b shows the preferred engineering design with the tensile triangles highlighting the rounded edges which are favorable in terms of a reduced stress concentration. A simple method in engineering design guides the clinical preparation.

Considering veneered zirconia or veneered glass-ceramic bridges, a finite element study

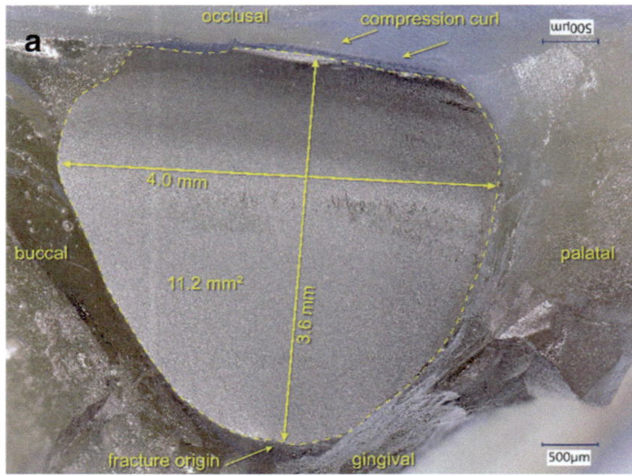

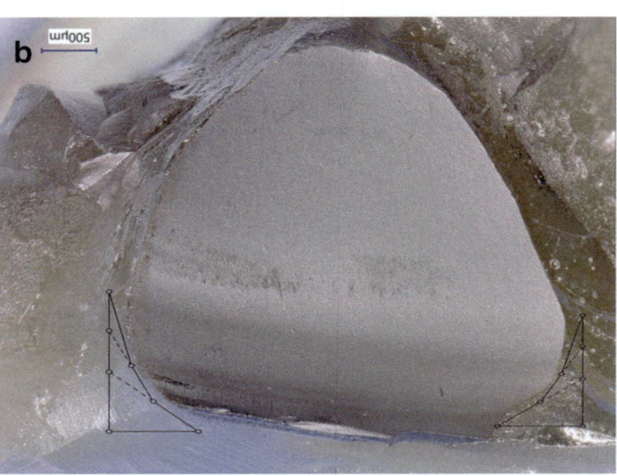

Fig. 5.29 A connector fracture of a posterior zirconia bridge in buccal-palatal direction, exhibiting a cross-sectional area of 11.2 mm² (**a**). This triangulated connector design would become more fracture resistant when simply rotating by 180° (**b**). The MTTs show the benefit from rounded angles (image by courtesy of Prof. S. Scherrer, Geneva, Switzerland)

investigated on substantial stress concentrations at the gingival side of the connector, located at the interface between core and veneer [50]. Apart from a higher stress concentration in zirconia veneered compared to glass-ceramic veneered frameworks, they concluded that the gingival notch radius of a connector in mesiodistal direction has a substantial influence on the fracture resistance. This is an important factor in engineering design of bridge connectors as pointed out by Quinn et al. [51]. Not only the connector cross-section but more relevant the notch factor at the gingival side of a connector in mesiodistal extension is limiting the fracture resistance. A greater radius of the gingiva curvature is desired with typical values ranging from $r = 0.2$ to $r = 0.5$ mm [51]. The mesiodistal radius is the critical design parameter when considering stress concentration and clinical fracture incidence. Taken from Fig. 4.13, Fig. 5.30 highlights this region and the tensile triangles show the preferred design preparing blunt notches, as they are oriented perpendicular to the applied tensile stress upon bending of a bridge.

The above onsiderations regarding stress distribution and notch effect in the connector regions however fail to holf for posterior two-unit cantilever bridge constructs. As the support

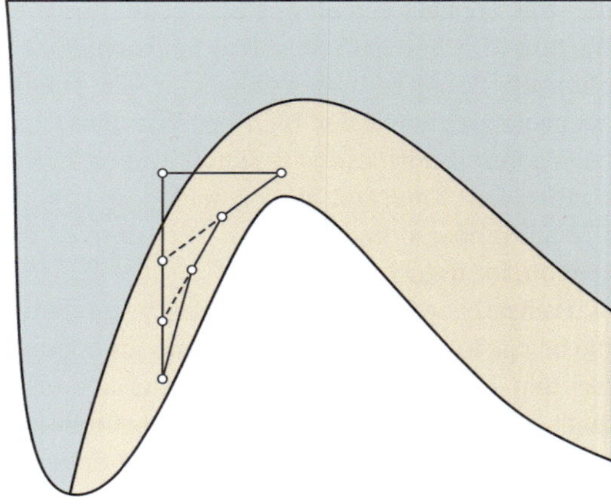

Fig. 5.30 Magnification from Fig. 4.13 shows the gingiva connector region in mesiodistal direction. The MTTs are guiding a preferred design with reduced stress concentration, by preparing a wider radius of the curvature

on the second abutment tooth is missing, the bending moment under occlusal, vertical load is no longer located at the gingiva side but highly stress concentrated on the occlusal side of the connector region. Numerical simulations of the two-unit cantilever bridge situation have identified the specific stress state and has proposed shape optimization for improved mechanical performance [52].

5.3.6   The Implant

Zirconia, specifically the 3Y-TZP subtype, became a suitable ceramic alternative to titanium or titanium alloys for manufacturing dental implants [53]. The clinical performance, osseointegration kinetics, mechanical fatigue stability, and long-term performance have been thoroughly investigated in recent years. Clinical studies and review summaries reported acceptable long-term performance for zirconia, in the majority of cases compared to established titanium implant materials [54]. However, certain clinical failure rates have been associated with implant fractures. Interestingly, the scientific approach in implant dentistry follows the proposed procedure of this book: learning from meticulous fractographic examination (destruction) and translating into clinical resistant and stable construction design [55–57], which is rarely found in restorative or prosthetic dentistry. Figure 5.31 shows examples of clinically fractured ceramic implants.

Those fractographic evidence is extremely valuable, as most fractures are related to weak construction design of ceramic implants as in the beginning, the construction principles valid for tough titanium were simply transferred to brittle ceramics. As the elastic modulus of titanium is half the modulus of zirconia while offering a ten times greater toughness, the material response and fracture resistance to external loading are widely different for both materials and cannot be linearly converted. Based on translational research studies, several regions of fracture susceptibility have been identified. Among others, there is the length to thickness ratio, various thread parameters, the implant surface, and the implant-abutment connection.

From an engineering perspective, the dental implant is an extremely complex compartment, consisting of the implant, the abutment and the prosthetic crown, together jointed by form fit or adhesive fit. Figure 5.32 shows a cross section through a zirconia implant.

Implant Length and Thickness

Thickness becomes a critical issue when replacing an anterior tooth with reduced bone support or due to esthetic reasons leading to selection of diameter reduced implants. A retrospective, forensic clinical study investigated on the reasons for fracture of diameter reduced (3.25 mm) ceramic implants in the anterior region [56]. Due to substantial bending moments in labial-oral direction, the implants fractured after 8–26 months, while the fracture origins were located at the first turn of the thread, i.e., at the bone crest level, as this is the location of the maximum bending moment.

The influence of variations in thickness and length on fracture resistance is a target research area for titanium as well as for ceramic implants. The central aim behind those investigations is to reduce the stress concentration at the interface

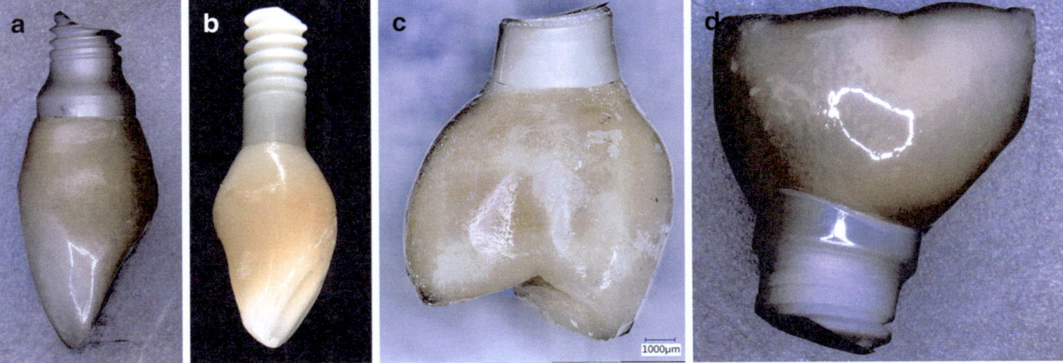

Fig. 5.31 Two anterior (**a**, **b**) and two posterior (**c**, **d**) examples of clinically fractured ceramic implants exhibiting the fracture plane at the first turn of the thread; Fig. 5.31b shows a deeper fracture plane due to extensive, marginal peri-implant bone loss (images by courtesy of Prof. S. Scherrer, Geneva, Switzerland [55])

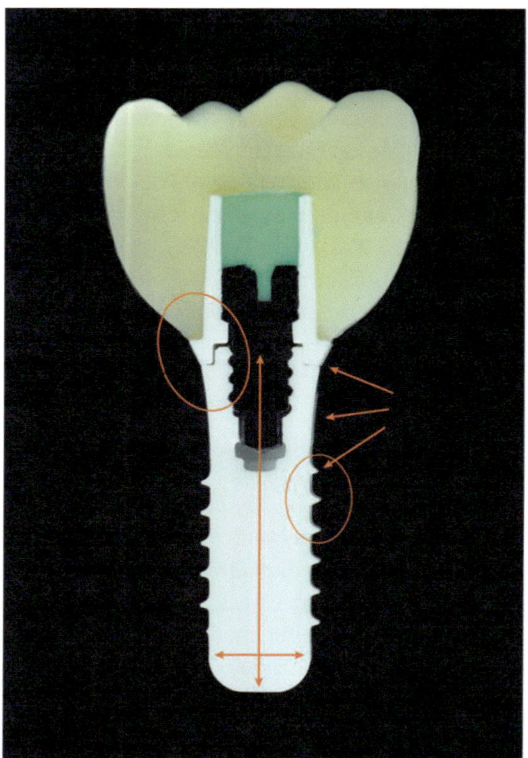

Fig. 5.32 Cross section through a restored ceramic implant (Zeramex P6, Dentalpoint AG; Switzerland, Ø 4.8 × 12 mm, ATZ (alumina toughened zirconia), straight abutment, resin composite molar crown). Regions of special attention are labelled in red: the length to thickness ratio, the thread design, the implant surface, and the implant-abutment connection

between the implant and the surrounding bone to a minimum, especially around the implant neck to the crestal bone. Finite element modelling showed a significant stress reduction at wider implant diameters [58–60]. Those in silico studies were calculated using titanium implant materials. Expanding those findings to zirconia as implant material, the effect is even amplified as titanium has an elastic modulus of 105 GPa compared to the stiffness of zirconia ($E = 200$ GPa) [53]. As a consequence, the notch effect of a reduced implant diameter is increasing the stress concentration at the interface to the surrounding bone, especially when using stiffer implant materials.

The bending moment, that is effective on the incisal edge of the anterior crown and maximized at the bone level is further dynamically influenced by marginal peri-implant bone loss over time [61]. Once a patient suffers from severe peri-implantitis, thereby decreasing the bone level, the maximum bending moment increases, too (see Fig. 5.31b).

Implant Thread Design

The design of the implant screw, namely the internal threads of the screw connection of a two-piece implant system and the external thread that connect with the surrounding tissue are further potential fracture sensitive locations. The external thread is exposed to torque moments during placement and to shear and bending moments during oral function [62]. A ceramic screw, in general, has to fulfill the same purpose as the metal analogon, as it has to cut and proceed into the surrounding substrate with minimum torque and has to fix the implant in position and resist against external forces. However, due to the far greater brittleness of ceramics, a design cannot be simply copied from established constructions for ductile metals.

Figure 5.33 schematically introduces the main characteristics of a thread. A thread is described by the root and the crest, defining the minor and the major diameter of the implant, the thread and the helix angles and the pitch, the distance between two crests. Thread parameters, such as, e.g., thread angle or helix angle are more relevant for cutting properties, while others, such as pitch or thread depth are more related to a stable construction.

In that context, the inner screw, that connects the implant to the abutment, is mainly under tension, holding both parts in intimate, frictional contact, while the external implant thread is under combined bending, shear, and compressive loading, as preset by the oral occlusal situation. An anterior implant is rather exposed to high shear and bending forces while the posterior implant is more under compressive and bending loading. The thread design has to account for the

Fig. 5.33 Principal characteristics of a thread

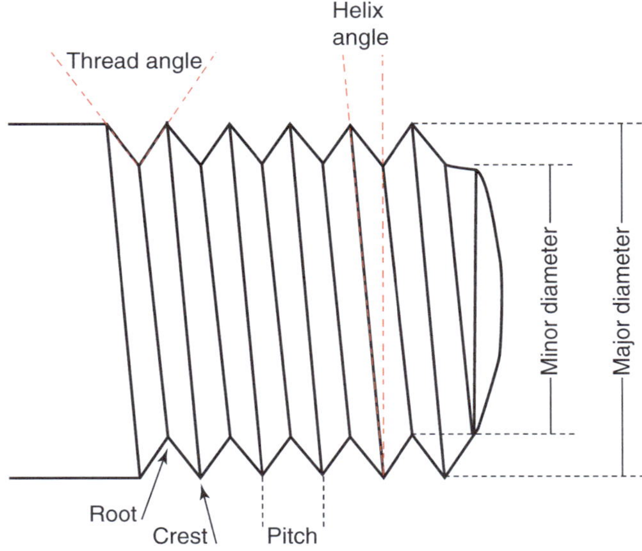

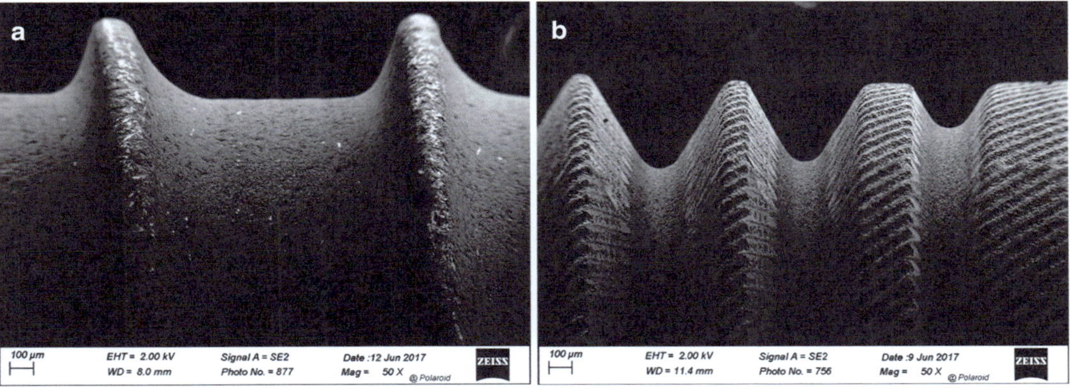

Fig. 5.34 Thread design of the Zeramex P6 implant system ((**a**); compare Fig. 5.32) and of the Zirkolith Z5m ((**b**); Z-Systems AG, Switzerland) implant (images by courtesy of Prof. S. Scherrer, Geneva, Switzerland)

specific application. Figure 5.34a shows an example of a ceramic thread design (from Fig. 5.32) with long pitches and comparably low thread depth combined with steep thread angles. A closer look shows us the slightly steeper bottom flanges compared to the upper flanges, as vertical occlusal loads are better absorbed by the plateau. Figure 5.34b shows the tapered, crestal part of a ceramic implant with an increasing minor diameter when reaching the connection of the thread with the implant body. The thread crests are textured to increase the frictional set of the implant.

Apart from the dental implant design, Fig. 5.35 shows a numeric simulation of an optimized ceramic thread, thereby visualizing the application of the MTT [25]. However, designed for a completely different engineering application, the structural optimization is closely matching the shape of the Zeramex P6 implant, as shown in Fig. 5.34a.

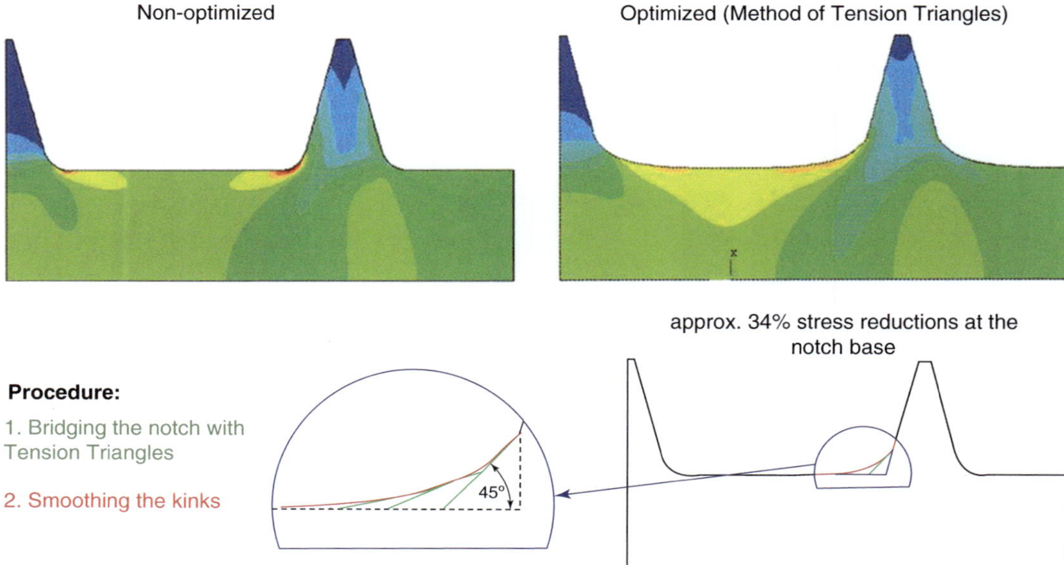

Fig. 5.35 Finite element structural optimization of a ceramic thread, visualizing the application of the MTT [25]

Implant-Abutment Connection

Ceramic implants were first introduced as one-piece implants combining the endosseous implant and the abutment in one single unit. This was mainly owed to improved stability and fracture resistance of the implant. With material improvements and clinical progress, also two-piece implants were designed and marketed [63, 64]. Therein, one critical step was to establish a tight connection between the abutment and the implant body. While for titanium implants, a conical, frictional connection was found beneficial, this would not hold for complex and filigree connections using brittle ceramics. According to the principle of converting tensile in compressive stress, the solution was to create a flat, tight platform that is connected by form fit, employing an internal screw (see Fig. 5.32). The abutment-implant connection on the one side has to provide sufficient strength against occlusal loads and on the other hand to establish a tight seal against oral microorganisms. In general, 3Y-TZP zirconia or ATZ showed sufficient strength as abutment material, but the key was still the complex construction design [53, 63]. The anti-rotational element of the connection requires space and sufficient wall thickness, not always provided by the various designs, such as triangle, hexagon, or octagon connections. Especially in dense bone sites, the torquing moment applied on the connector fit of the endosseous implant might overload a weakly designed connection [57].

Mechanical stability and fatigue resistance of the implant-abutment connection is commonly approached in combined in vitro and in silico studies. The standardized ISO 14801 dynamic loading test for endosseous implants has been established to dynamically load an implant under certain angulations [65]. The use of finite element modelling in combination with structural optimization (CAO) thereby assists in designing the optimum connector type [61, 66].

Implant Surface

Apart from the implant macrodesign, the microdesign or texture of the ceramic surface substantially influences the fracture resistance. On the one side, a retentive and coarse surface roughness offering a large surface area is said to act beneficial in terms of optimized osseointegration [67]. On the other side, a coarse roughness is a critical source for fracture releasing defects. While the optimum roughness for osseointegration is still under controversial scientific discussion, the benefit from a smooth, defect-free surface is clearly providing maximum fracture strength. This trade-off situation has to be carefully assessed and a small window of application guides the implant surface microdesign. Especially the junction between the thread and the implant body is of special attention as this is an exposed fracture site. The thread region needs the surface roughness for osseointegration while a polished surface at the implant neck prevents biofilm adsorption and plaque formation. The influence of zirconia surface defects has been shown in fractography supported clinical research on fractured implants [68]. Among other sources, damaging surface treatment or machining defects have been identified as reasons for fracture.

A gentle grit-blasting strategy or improved coating procedures might help reducing the critical surface defects and hence accounting for a reliable implant microdesign. The choice of a different material offering improved fracture resistance is further recommended. Alumina toughened zirconia (ATZ) might be a suitable solution for improvement [69]. This material has long been used for arthoplastic prostheses. It has been shown that ATZ offers a fracture toughness of K_{Ic} = 5–6 MPa.m$^{0.5}$ and a fracture strength of 1800–2400 MPa [70]. The choice of a material with improved fatigue resistance and stability against low-temperature degradation is a further option for improvement.

References

1. Posselt U, Andersen A. Studies in the mobility of the human mandible. Copenhagen; 1952.
2. Posselt U. Physiology of occlusion and rehabilitation. Oxford: Blackwell Scientific; 1968.
3. Buschang PH, Hayasaki H, Throckmorton GS. Quantification of human chewing-cycle kinematics. Arch Oral Biol. 2000;45(6):461–74.
4. Proschel P, Hofmann M. Frontal chewing patterns of the incisor point and their dependence on resistance of food and type of occlusion. J Prosthet Dent. 1988;59(5):617–24.
5. Wiens JP. Fundamentals of occlusion. Chicago: American College of Prosthodontists; 2015.
6. The glossary of prosthodontic terms: ninth edition. J Prosthet Dent. 2017;117(5S):e1–e105.
7. van der Bilt A, Engelen L, Pereira LJ, van der Glas HW, Abbink JH. Oral physiology and mastication. Physiol Behav. 2006;89(1):22–7.
8. Utz K-H. The tactile subtle sensibility of natural teeth—a clinical experimental research [Dissertation]. Bonn: Rheinische Friedrich-Wilhelms-Universität Bonn; 2014.
9. Wenz HJ, Hellwig E. Zahnärztliche Propädeutik. 14th ed. Cologne: Deutscher Ärzte-Verlag; 2018.
10. Rohrle O, Saini H, Ackland DC. Occlusal loading during biting from an experimental and simulation point of view. Dent Mater. 2018;34(1):58–68.
11. Martinez Choy SE, Lenz J, Schweizerhof K, Schmitter M, Schindler HJ. Realistic kinetic loading of the jaw system during single chewing cycles: a finite element study. J Oral Rehabil. 2017;44(5):375–84.
12. Bergmann G, Gandini R, Ruder H. Averaging of strongly varying signals. Biomed Tech (Berl). 2001;46(6):168–71.
13. Peck CC. Biomechanics of occlusion—implications for oral rehabilitation. J Oral Rehabil. 2016;43(3):205–14.
14. Schroeder HE. The periodontium. Heidelberg: Springer; 1986.
15. Lang NP, Lindhe J. Clinical periodontology and implant dentistry. 6th ed. Hoboken: Wiley-Blackwell; 2015.
16. Haraldson T. Comparisons of chewing patterns in patients with bridges supported on osseointegrated implants and subjects with natural dentitions. Acta Odontol Scand. 1983;41(4):203–8.
17. He LH, Fujisawa N, Swain MV. Elastic modulus and stress–strain response of human enamel by nanoindentation. Biomaterials. 2006;27(24):4388–98.
18. Kinney JH, Balooch M, Marshall GW, Marshall SJ. A micromechanics model of the elastic properties of human dentine. Arch Oral Biol. 1999;44(10):813–22.
19. Roesler J, Harders H, Baeker M. Mechanical behaviour of engineering materials. Berlin: Springer; 2007.
20. Darvell BW. Materials science for dentistry. Oxford: Woodhead; 2018.
21. Mattheck C. The face of failure in nature and engineering. Karlsruhe: Karlsruhe Institute of Technology; 2004.
22. ISO 6872:2015. Dentistry—ceramic materials. Geneva: International Organization for Standardization; 2015.
23. Wendler M, Kaizer MR, Belli R, Lohbauer U, Zhang Y. Sliding contact wear and subsurface damage of CAD/CAM materials against zirconia. Dent Mater. 2020;36(3):387–401.
24. Mattheck C. Pauli explains the form in nature. Karlsruhe: Karlsruhe Institute of Technology; 2018.
25. Mattheck C. Thinking tools after nature. Karlsruhe: Karlsruhe Institute of Technology; 2011.
26. ISO 18459:2015. Biomimetics—biomimetic structural optimization. Geneva: International Organization for Standardization; 2015.

27. Mattheck C, Kappel R, Kraft O. Meaning of the 45°-angle in mechanical design according to nature. WIT Trans Ecol Environ. 2008;114:139–46.

28. Mattheck C, Greiner C, Bethge K, Tesari I, Weber K. The force cone method applied to explain hidden whirls in tribology. Materials. 2021;14(14):3894.

29. Berkovitz BKB, Boyde A, Frank RM, Höhling HJ, Moxham BJ, Nalbandian J, et al. Teeth. Berlin: Springer; 1989.

30. Bechtle S, Habelitz S, Klocke A, Fett T, Schneider GA. The fracture behaviour of dental enamel. Biomaterials. 2010;31(2):375–84.

31. Belli R, Petschelt A, Lohbauer U. Thermal-induced residual stresses affect the fractographic patterns of zirconia-veneer dental prostheses. J Mech Behav Biomed Mater. 2013;21:167–77.

32. Wan BY, Shahmoradi M, Zhang ZP, Shibata Y, Sarrafpour B, Swain M, et al. Modelling of stress distribution and fracture in dental occlusal fissures. Sci Rep. 2019;9:4682.

33. Couegnat G, Fok SL, Cooper JE, Qualtrough AJ. Structural optimization of dental restorations using the principle of adaptive growth. Dent Mater. 2006;22(1):3–12.

34. Belli R, Wendler M, de Ligny D, Cicconi MR, Petschelt A, Peterlik H, et al. Chairside CAD/CAM materials. Part 1: measurement of elastic constants and microstructural characterization. Dent Mater. 2017;33(1):84–98.

35. Kelly RJ. Ceramics in dentistry: principles and practice. Hanover Park, IL: Quintessence; 2016.

36. Hsueh CH, Miranda P. Modeling of contact-induced radial cracking in ceramic bilayer coatings on compliant substrates. J Mater Res. 2003;18(5):1275–83.

37. Shahmoradi M, Wan B, Zhang Z, Wilson T, Swain M, Li Q. Monolithic crowns fracture analysis: the effect of material properties, cusp angle and crown thickness. Dent Mater. 2020;36(8):1038–51.

38. Belli R, Petschelt A, Hofner B, Hajto J, Scherrer SS, Lohbauer U. Fracture rates and lifetime estimations of CAD/CAM all-ceramic restorations. J Dent Res. 2016;95(1):67–73.

39. Oilo M, Gjerdet NR. Fractographic analyses of all-ceramic crowns: a study of 27 clinically fractured crowns. Dent Mater. 2013;29(6):e78–84.

40. Oilo M, Kvam K, Tibballs JE, Gjerdet NR. Clinically relevant fracture testing of all-ceramic crowns. Dent Mater. 2013;29(8):815–23.

41. Belli R, Volkl H, Csato S, Tremmel S, Wartzack S, Lohbauer U. Development of a hoop-strength test for model sphero-cylindrical dental ceramic crowns: FEA and fractography. J Eur Ceram Soc. 2020;40(14):4753–64.

42. Preis V, Dowerk T, Behr M, Kolbeck C, Rosentritt M. Influence of cusp inclination and curvature on the in vitro failure and fracture resistance of veneered zirconia crowns. Clin Oral Investig. 2014;18(3):891–900.

43. Kirsten A, Parkot D, Raith S, Fischer H. A cusp supporting framework design can decrease critical stresses in veneered molar crowns. Dent Mater. 2014;30(3):321–6.

44. Lohbauer U, Scherrer SS, Della Bona A, Tholey M, van Noort R, Vichi A, et al. ADM guidance-ceramics: all-ceramic multilayer interfaces in dentistry. Dent Mater. 2017;33(6):585–98.

45. Tuntiprawon M, Wilson PR. The effect of cement thickness on the fracture strength of all-ceramic crowns. Aust Dent J. 1995;40(1):17–21.

46. Yu H, Chen YH, Cheng H, Sawase T. Finish-line designs for ceramic crowns: a systematic review and meta-analysis. J Prosthet Dent. 2019;122(1):22–30 e5.

47. Larsson C. Zirconium dioxide based dental restorations. Studies on clinical performance and fracture behaviour. Swed Dent J Suppl. 2011;213:9–84.

48. Takuma Y, Nomoto S, Sato T, Sugihara N. Effect of framework design on fracture resistance in zirconia 4-unit all-ceramic fixed partial dentures. Bull Tokyo Dent Coll. 2013;54(3):149–56.

49. Murase T, Nomoto S, Sato T, Shinya A, Koshihara T, Yasuda H. Effect of connector design on fracture resistance in all-ceramic fixed partial dentures for mandibular incisor region. Bull Tokyo Dent Coll. 2014;55(3):149–55.

50. Lin J, Shinya A, Gomi H, Shinya A. Finite element analysis to compare stress distribution of connector of lithia disilicate-reinforced glass-ceramic and zirconia-based fixed partial denture. Odontology. 2012;100(1):96–9.

51. Quinn GD, Studart AR, Hebert C, VerHoef JR, Arola D. Fatigue of zirconia and dental bridge geometry: design implications. Dent Mater. 2010;26(12):1133–6.

52. Shi L, Fok AS. Structural optimization of the fibre-reinforced composite substructure in a three-unit dental bridge. Dent Mater. 2009;25(6):791–801.

53. Osman RB, Swain MV. A critical review of dental implant materials with an emphasis on titanium versus zirconia. Materials. 2015;8(3):932–58.

54. Osman RB, Swain MV. A critical review of dental implant materials with an emphasis on titanium versus zirconia. Materials (Basel). 2015;8(3):932–58.

55. Scherrer SS, Mekki M, Crottaz C, Gahlert M, Romelli E, Marger L, et al. Translational research on clinically failed zirconia implants. Dent Mater. 2019;35(2):368–88.

56. Gahlert M, Burtscher D, Grunert I, Kniha H, Steinhauser E. Failure analysis of fractured dental zirconia implants. Clin Oral Implants Res. 2012;23(3):287–93.

57. Osman RB, Ma S, Duncan W, De Silva RK, Siddiqi A, Swain MV. Fractured zirconia implants and related implant designs: scanning electron microscopy analysis. Clin Oral Implants Res. 2013;24(5):592–7.

58. Huang S-C, Tsai C-F. Finite element analysis of a dental implant. Biomed Eng. 2003;15(2):82–5.

59. El-Anwar MI, El-Zawahry MM. A three dimensional finite element study on dental implant design. J Genet Eng Biotechnol. 2011;9(1):77–82.

60. Himmlova L, Dostalova T, Kacovsky A, Konvickova S. Influence of implant length and diameter on stress distribution: a finite element analysis. J Prosthet Dent. 2004;91(1):20–5.
61. Streckbein P, Streckbein RG, Wilbrand JF, Malik CY, Schaaf H, Howaldt HP, et al. Non-linear 3D evaluation of different oral implant-abutment connections. J Dent Res. 2012;91(12):1184–9.
62. Scherrer SS, Cesar PF, Lohbauer U, Belli R. Zirconia as a biomaterial in implant dentistry. Forum Implant. 2018;14(1):6–17.
63. Nakamura K, Kanno T, Milleding P, Ortengren U. Zirconia as a dental implant abutment material: a systematic review. Int J Prosthodont. 2010;23(4):299–309.
64. Gomes AL, Montero J. Zirconia implant abutments: a review. Med Oral Patol Oral Cir Bucal. 2011;16(1):e50–5.
65. ISO:14801. Dentistry—implants—dynamic loading test for endosseous dental implants. Geneva: International Organization for Standardization; 2016.
66. Ziębowicz B, Ziębowicz A, Baczkowski B, Kajzer W, Kajzer A. Biomechanical analysis of individual all-ceramic abutments used in dental implantology. Arch Metall Mater. 2016;61(3):1011–6.
67. Albrektsson T, Wennerberg A. On osseointegration in relation to implant surfaces. Clin Implant Dent Relat Res. 2019;21(Suppl 1):4–7.
68. Osman RB, Ma SY, Duncan W, De Silva RK, Siddiqi A, Swain MV. Fractured zirconia implants and related implant designs: scanning electron microscopy analysis. Clin Oral Implan Res. 2013;24(5):592–7.
69. Piconi C, Maccauro G. Zirconia as a ceramic biomaterial. Biomaterials. 1999;20(1):1–25.
70. Pabst W, Havrda J, Gregorova E, Krcmova B. Alumina toughened zirconia made by room temperature extrusion of ceramic pastes. Ceram-Silikaty. 2000;44(2):41–7.

Correction to: Construction Prevents Destruction

Correction to:
Chapter 5 in: U. Lohbauer and R. Belli, *Dental Ceramics*
https://doi.org/10.1007/978-3-030-94687-6_5

This original version of chapter 5 was inadvertently published with the incorrect figure 5.23. This chapter has been updated with the correct figure and legend on page 113.

Incorrect figure 5.23

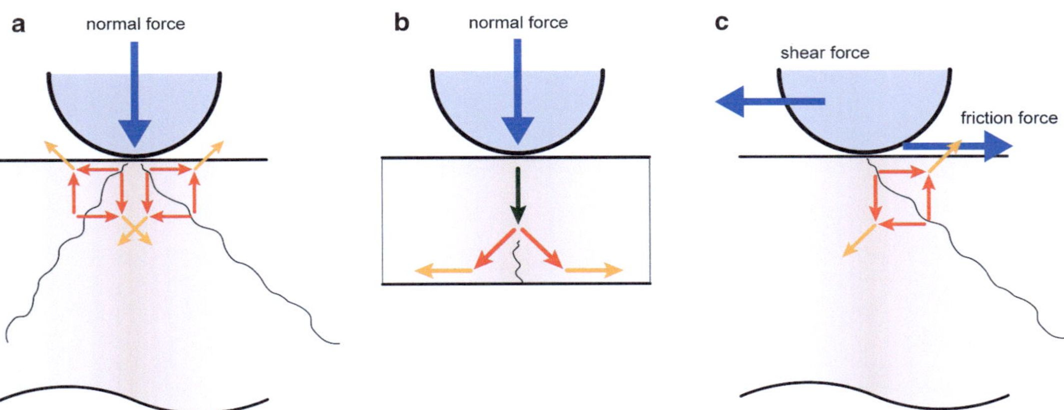

Fig. 5.23 Principle understanding of occlusal contact point mechanics under normal versus shear forces showing the development of internal tensile stress and hence a likely direction of crack propagation upon overloading. While Hertzian contacts upon normal loading tend to initiate cone cracks starting at the contact zone (**a**); the contact in thin plates (as found is weakly supported or thin restorations) follows the bending configuration respective crack profiles (**b**). Under shear loading (**c**), the stress is counteracted by the frictional resistance (e.g., upon severe bruxing) and a cone type of crack propagates behind the contact

The updated original version of the chapter can be found at https://doi.org/10.1007/978-3-030-94687-6_5

Correct figure 5.23

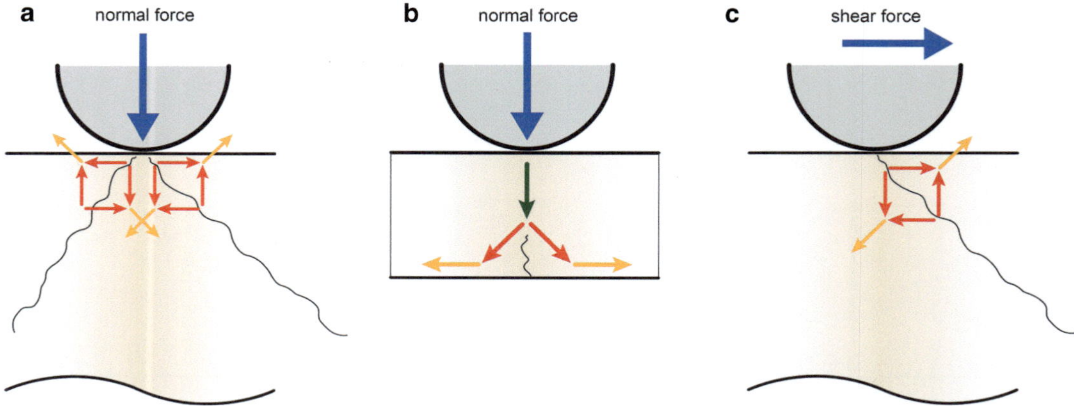

Fig. 5.23 Principle understanding of occlusal contact point mechanics under normal and shear forces showing the development of internal tensile stress and hence a likely direction of crack propagation upon overloading. While Hertzian contacts upon normal loading tend to initiate cone cracks starting at the contact zone (**a**), the contact in thin plates (as found is weakly supported or thin restorations) follows the bending configuration respective crack profiles (**b**). Under shear loading (**c**), the Hertzian pressure (e.g., upon severe bruxing) induces a cone type of crack that propagates ahead of the contact pressure zone

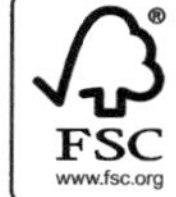